General Practice Cases
at a Glance

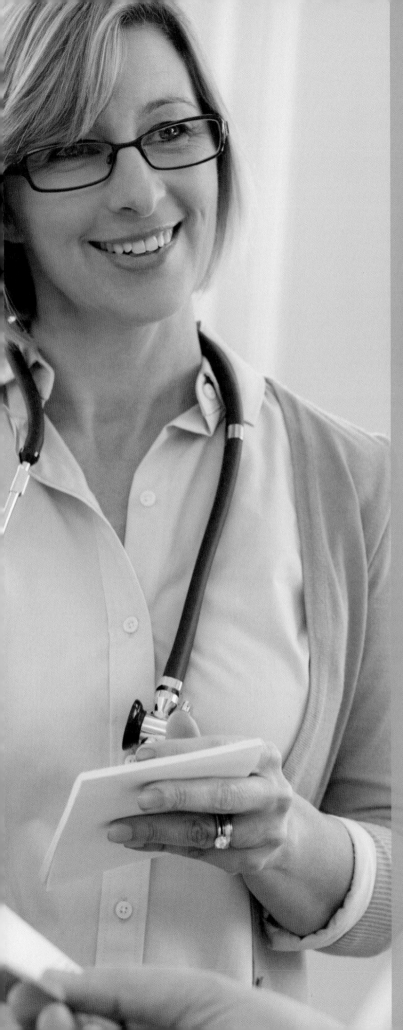

General Practice Cases

at a Glance

Carol Cooper

Honorary Teaching Fellow
Department of Primary Care and Public Health
Imperial College London
General Practitioner
London, UK

Martin Block

Programme Director
Imperial GP Specialty Training
Department of Primary Care and Public Health
Imperial College London
GP Partner, Clapham Park Group Practice
London, UK

WILEY Blackwell

Library of Congress Cataloging-in-Publication Data
Names: Cooper, Carol, 1951- , author. | Block, Martin (General practitioner), author.
    Title: General practice cases at a glance / Carol Cooper, Martin Block.
    Other titles: At a glance series (Oxford, England)
    Description: Chichester, West Sussex ; Malden, MA : John Wiley & Sons Inc., 2016. | Series: At a glance | Includes bibliographical references and index.
    Identifiers: LCCN 2015045693 | ISBN 9781119043782 (pbk.)
    Subjects: | MESH: General Practice—methods—Case Reports. | General Practice—methods—Problems and Exercises.
    Classification: LCC RC46 | NLM WB 18.2 | DDC 616—dc23
    LC record available at http://lccn.loc.gov/2015045693

A catalogue record for this book is available from the British Library.

Wiley also publishes its books in a variety of electronic formats. Some content that appears in print may not be available in electronic books.

Cover image: © Hero Images/Getty

Set in 9.5/11.5pt Minion Pro by Aptara Inc., New Delhi, India
Printed and bound in Singapore by Markono Print Media Pte Ltd

1 2017

Contents

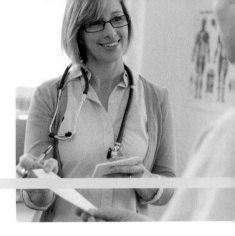

Preface   vii

Part 1

Introduction   1

1   The consultation   2
2   Clinical reasoning to reach a diagnosis   4

Part 2

Cases   7

1   My baby is burning up   8
2   I need something for hay fever   10
3   I can't seem to shift this cough   12
4   My knee is very bad   14
5   I have migraine   16
6   I've come for my flu jab   18
7   He's a little terror   20
8   I've got a problem with my shoulder   22
9   I can't believe how much weight I've put on   24
10   It's my back passage   26
11   I am pregnant again   28
12   My baby has an upset tummy   30
13   My ear really hurts   32
14   I'm worried about my drinking   33
15   She cries all the time   34
16   I need something to help me sleep   36
17   My eye hurts   38
18   I think I should get this prostate test, doctor   40
19   I can't live with this pain much longer   41
20   I've got a red eye   44
21   I'm fed up with my spots   46
22   I've come for the results of my blood tests   48
23   I'd like to talk to you about HRT   50
24   I've got a bit of a discharge   52
25   I'm feeling tired and woozy   54
26   I think I need to get my blood pressure checked   56
27   Well, I'm pregnant   58
28   I've been feeling short of breath   60
29   She's coughing non-stop   62
30   I'm worried about my memory   64
31   I've got this pain in my chest, doctor   66
32   I've been having terrible stomach cramps   68
33   I'm concerned this mole has been growing   70
34   I seem to have lost weight   72

35   I'm worried about my erection   74

36   I think the cancer has got me   76

37   I'm all over the place these days   78

38   She's had tummy ache for two days   80

39   I don't want to have my period when I am on holiday   82

40   It's my leg   84

41   I'm having terrible diarrhoea   86

42   The nurse did my diabetes check last week.
         I'm here for the results   88

43   My skin is really itchy   90

44   Doctor, I'm just feeling really down   92

45   I've got a really bad burning in my stomach   93

46   I want to talk about my risk of breast cancer   94

47   I've got a terrible back ache   96

48   I'd like antibiotics please   98

49   I'm tired all the time   100

50   I'm worried about this lump, doctor   102

List of abbreviations   105
Index of cases by speciality   106
Index   107

Preface

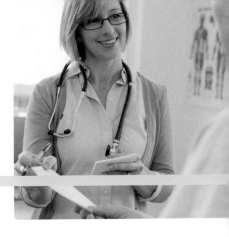

General practice has seen huge changes in the last few years and is on course for many more. Areas once considered the exclusive province of secondary care have shifted to primary care.

The consultation is at the heart of general practice: a one-to-one exchange (unless there are relatives in tow) where the GP can assess the problem, make a working diagnosis, and plan management with the patient. It's a lot to do in just 10 or 15 minutes.

This makes the GP attachment the ideal place for a medical student to learn essential skills, like focused history-taking, examination, clinical decision-making and good communication. Even if you ultimately choose to work in a speciality very unlike general practice, you will find these skills useful.

The book is by two practising GPs who are linked with the academic department of primary care at London's Imperial College Medical School. It is a companion volume to *General Practice at a Glance*, but can be used on its own.

These 50 consultations cover all age ranges and a broad spread of clinical areas. Some you could consider 'bread-and-butter general practice', while others contain less common conditions that shouldn't be missed. The book follows the 'at a Glance' style: clear and concise, with charts and tables to accompany each case, and clinical guidelines to make sure students are up to speed with current thinking.

Every scenario is symptom-based, because that's how patients present. The cases reflect the diversity of today's patient population as well as the spread of common symptoms. Each begins with a short opening quote such as, 'I am tired all the time'.

With each one, you'll have to tease out the relevant history, decide what to examine and which investigations are needed, reach a working diagnosis and formulate a management plan. You will be put on the spot, just as in your exams, and just as you will be in real-life clinical practice.

While the patients are fictionalized, they are complex and realistic, and, as in everyday medicine, some provide lighter moments too.

Each case takes one or two pages and includes:
- the history, including a brief PMH and current medication
- questions for you to answer as you go along
- red flag symptoms and signs which mustn't be missed (marked ▶)
- useful info, charts and graphics
- further resources, mostly online, to deepen your knowledge.

We suggest you ask yourself at the end of every case, 'What have I learnt here?'

You can work your way through the book, or dip in wherever you want. The consultations are arranged randomly, to reflect clinical general practice. However the index can guide you to consultations system by system for revision purposes if you like.

We wrote this title to:
- reflect the richness of general practice
- challenge students to think on their feet
- make them commit their thoughts
- enable them get the most from their general practice attachment
- give them tools to become good doctors.

We hope you enjoy this book and wish you success and fulfillment in your career.

Carol Cooper
Martin Block

Disclaimer

Patients in this book are designed to reflect real life, with their own reports of symptoms and concerns. Please note that all names used are entirely fictitious and any similarity to individuals, alive or dead, is coincidental.

Acknowledgements

Martin: I would like to offer thanks to my trainees past and present and to Anna Strhan for her support and constant inspiration.

Carol: I would like to thank my colleagues Paul Booton, Graham Easton, Rob Hicks and Sally Mason, and my students at Imperial College.

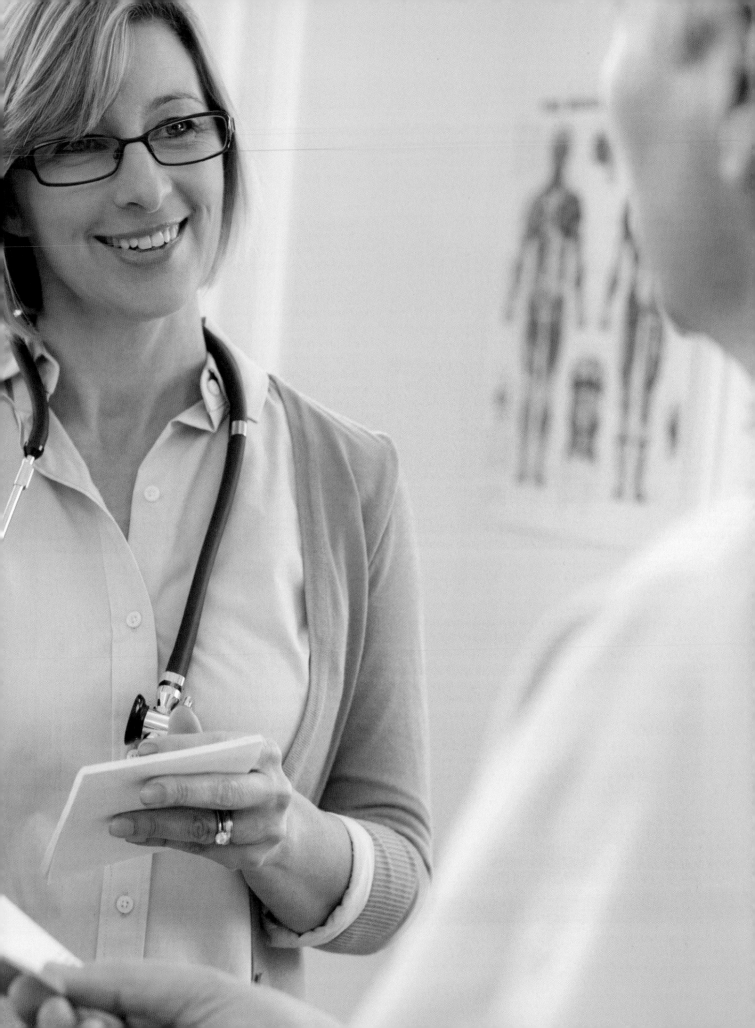

Introduction

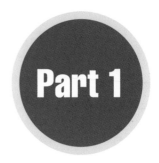

Part 1

Chapters

1   The consultation   2
2   Clinical reasoning to reach a diagnosis   4

1 The consultation

The vast majority of medical care takes place in general practice, with well over 300 million consultations a year in the UK. That makes general practice the first port of call for every symptom you can imagine, and then some. For many patients, it is the only port of call. So it's imperative to get the consultation right.

In general practice, you'll find a microcosm of all the clinical specialities, and there's no way of knowing what will come in next. All the consultations in this book take place in general practice, either in practice premises or at home, but good consultation skills lie at the heart of good medicine in every field, whether you are a GP or a neurosurgeon. Use your time in general practice wisely and make sure you learn these eminently transferrable skills.

While textbooks are usually disease based, consultations are patient based, most often around a presenting symptom. Teasing out what is wrong requires **focused history-taking** and **clinical reasoning**. In time these will become second nature to you, and you will also get faster as you become more experienced.

Some consultations may be straightforward. Others much less so, and your patient may need more than one consultation to do the problem justice.

Focused history-taking vs. traditional history-taking

A traditional medical history is very complete, usually proceeds in a structured way, and takes a long time because it leaves no stone unturned. It is the best way to learn when starting your clinical studies, but not always appropriate for every problem. If your patient has acute chest pain, it is hardly relevant to know if her mother had arthritis – and going into such detail will delay treatment.

A focused history demands clinical judgment as to what to delve into and what to leave. You may want to explore your patient's eye symptoms in depth, for instance, and ask few or no questions about his bowels and bladder.

How to take a focused history

• Open with a **general question** like, 'What can I do for you today?' and then listen attentively.

• Use the **'golden minute'**: give your patient time to open up about the problem without firing questions.
• Use **active listening.**
• Begin with **open questions,** followed by **closed questions**.

Open and closed questions

Open questions are useful at the beginning of your history taking. They give the patient space to give you important information. You can also use them to ask about how the symptoms are affecting your patient's life, what his mood is like and so on.

Closed questions are useful when you need to be clear about a specific detail. In general this is useful later in your history taking. For instance you might want to clarify a particular diagnosis (e.g. 'Is it worse when you breathe in?') or exclude a red flag (e.g. 'Have you seen any blood in your stool?').

Using mostly open questions, and then moving to a handful of appropriate closed questions helps GPs gain lots of information in a time-efficient way.

Tip

When you are next sitting in with a GP look out for when he or she asks open and closed questions.

Clarify what your patient tells you.
• 'What do you mean by *locking*?' Patients may also misuse medical terms, such as pernicious anaemia, and misquote the names of drugs they have taken.
• Be curious in your probing, but don't take statements for granted. 'I don't smoke,' may mean your patient stopped two weeks ago, fearing he has lung cancer.
Find out more about the symptoms.
• 'How often do you get up at night to pass water?'
• If there's pain, get the details. You could use **SOCRATES** (Site, Onset, Character, Radiation, Associated factors, Timing, Exacerbating/relieving factors, Severity on a scale of 0–10) (Figure 1.1).
• You can avoid an interrogative style by appropriate body language (e.g. smiling, nodding) to show a genuine interest in your patient.

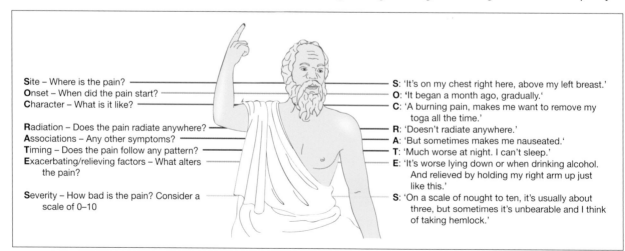

Figure 1.1 Using SOCRATES as a guide to taking a history.

General Practice Cases at a Glance, First Edition. Carol Cooper and Martin L Block. © 2017 John Wiley & Sons, Ltd. Published 2017 by John Wiley & Sons, Ltd.

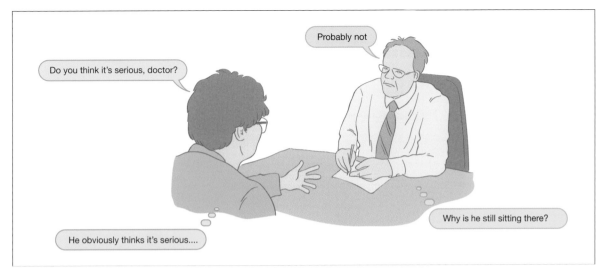

Figure 1.2 Ideas, concerns and expectations.

It is equally important to find out about **function**. What does the pain – or other symptoms – prevent your patient from doing? You will need to know something about his daily life, at work and at home, to make a judgement as to how bad it all is.

This is the place to ask some **red flag questions** to pick up or rule out serious conditions. 'Have you ever passed blood when you wee?'

Explore your patient's ideas, concerns and expectations (ICE)

Try questions like, 'What were you hoping I could do?', 'What are your thoughts on all this?' and 'What are you most worried about?' (Figure 1.2). Unless you ask, you may never know.

Use sign-posting

Summarize to let the patient know you're on the right wavelength. 'So let me see: your periods have been heavier for six months, and you've had a discharge that is mostly yellow and doesn't itch. Have I got it right?' It can also be a useful way of clarifying symptoms in your own mind.

Remember the **previous medical history** (PMH), including medication history, and recreational drugs and alcohol.

Family history is often relevant. Even if your patient doesn't have a familial problem, knowing the family history is a good pointer to what might be on his mind.

Examining the patient

Examination is equally important. If you don't examine the patient, you may as well judge a book by its cover. The general gist might be obvious, but you can't predict how the story might unfold. You need to strike a balance between a comprehensive physical examination, or a limited but well judged foray into one or two systems. However, don't cut corners. Always perform the examination your patient needs.

Think on your feet

Asking yourself, **'What next?'** This is part of the transition from student to doctor, and a hallmark of clinical responsibility. There's more on clinical reasoning in Chapter 2.

Share your thoughts with your patient. Your idea of treatment may not chime with his.

People skills

This book can't teach you bedside manners, but they're vital to building a rapport with your patient. Even if you are rushed, overworked or overwhelmed, patients deserve to see your courteous side.

Introductions are important. Before you ask what you can do for your patient today, give your name. A **smile** also does a huge amount to boost your patient's confidence and help concordance too.

Use appropriate **body language**, and a demeanour that shows your patient he has your full attention, at least for the next 10 minutes.

Resources and references

Books

Booton P, Cooper C, Easton G and Harper M. *General Practice at a Glance*. London: Wiley-Blackwell, 2013.

Douglas G, Nicol F and Robertson C. (eds.) *Macleod's Clinical Examination*. London: Elsevier, 2005.

Stephenson A. (ed.) *A Textbook of General Practice*. London: Hodder Arnold, 2004.

Fraser RC. (ed) *Clinical Method: a General Practice approach*. London: Butterworth Heinemann, 1999.

Neighbour R. *The Inner Consultation*. 2nd edn. Oxford: Radcliffe Publishing, 2004.

Silverman J, Kurtz S and Draper J. *Skills for Communicating with Patients*. Oxford: Radcliffe Medical Press, 2004.

Very comprehensive and reviews all the supporting research evidence.

Tate P. *The Doctor's Communication Handbook*. 5th edn. Oxford: Radcliffe Medical Press, 2006.

Articles

Almond S, Mant D and Thomson M. Diagnostic safety-netting. *Br J Gen Pract*. 2009; 59(568): 872–874.
http://bjgp.org/content/59/568/872

Henegan C. Diagnostic strategies used in primary care. *BMJ*. 2009; 338: 1003–1008.
http://www.bmj.com/content/338/bmj.b946

Clinical reasoning to reach a diagnosis

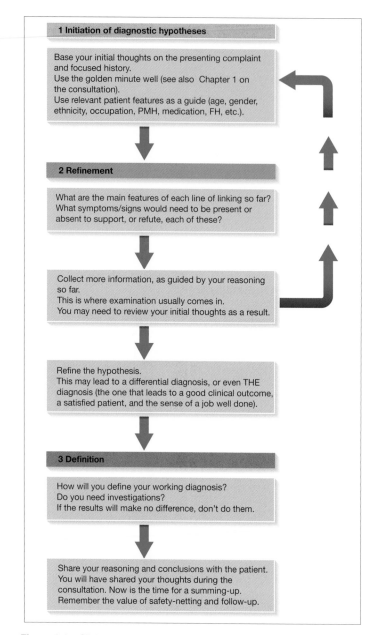

Figure 2.1 Clinical reasoning stages.

General Practice Cases at a Glance, First Edition. Carol Cooper and Martin L Block. © 2017 John Wiley & Sons, Ltd. Published 2017 by John Wiley & Sons, Ltd.

All doctors use clinical reasoning, but they rarely stop to think how they go through the process.

According to Henegan and others, clinical reasoning can be split into three stages:
* **initiation of a diagnostic hypothesis (or several)**
* **refinement of these**
* **definition of the final diagnosis**.

This is called the hypothetico-deductive model.

Initiation stage

The **initiation stage** usually coincides with the history, but can go on longer than that. The trigger for making your working hypothesis might be a **spot diagnosis**, as in the typical appearance of a BCC, or when you hear an opening snap. Or you might use the patient's **initial complaint** (say abdominal pain or sore throat) to guide your hypothesis making. On occasion you may even rely on the **patient's own diagnosis**. Self-labelling by patients always needs to be clarified during the consultation, so don't take it at face value. But it's not always wrong, either: think of pregnancy, or UTI. When making a hypothesis, another important trigger is **pattern recognition**. For instance weight gain, irregular periods and increasing facial hair should prompt thoughts of polycystic ovary syndrome.

If you don't have initial diagnostic thoughts, try to **name the problem**. In doing so, think of what might be causing it. This should generate some possibilities. Remember to take your patient's age, gender, occupation and past history into account. Also think of the **worst-case scenario**. This may be statistically rare, but it needs to be considered in every consultation. Otherwise you may miss important conditions.

Refinement stage

The next stage is **refinement**. Every scientific hypothesis is testable. Think of what you need to verify your theories so far. What are the questions you need to ask to support or oppose your hypotheses? And what clinical findings could you elicit either for or against your hypotheses? This will guide your next steps.

Reflect at every stage

* Is there anything you can't explain? Patients do sometimes have symptoms that don't conform to the textbook description, but beware of shoe-horning the facts to fit your preferred diagnosis.
* Consider too what the patient thinks, and their ICE (see Chapter 1 on the consultation).
* Don't discard the other possibilities or pigeon-hole your patient's problem too soon. **Errors of bias** can be serious.

Make sure you rule out important, rare, but serious possibilities. Here **red flags**, either in the history or the examination, can help. Remember there may be further red flags later, when any investigations come back.

Make use of **clinical decision-making tools**, if appropriate, like the Ottawa ankle rules or the International Prostate Symptom Score. You'll find other tools in this book too.

Ask yourself, 'Is this patient ill?' It's especially apt when seeing a child, but applies to most clinical situations. This may clarify your thinking, as well as determine the degree of urgency.

The **final definition phase** can include further tests, a trial of treatment, or discussion with a colleague. If you can't make a diagnosis now, consider whether a diagnosis needs to be made this minute, or whether it can wait. Reviewing the patient in a few days, or a week, may allow time for the natural history of the condition to evolve, although this is obviously not always appropriate.

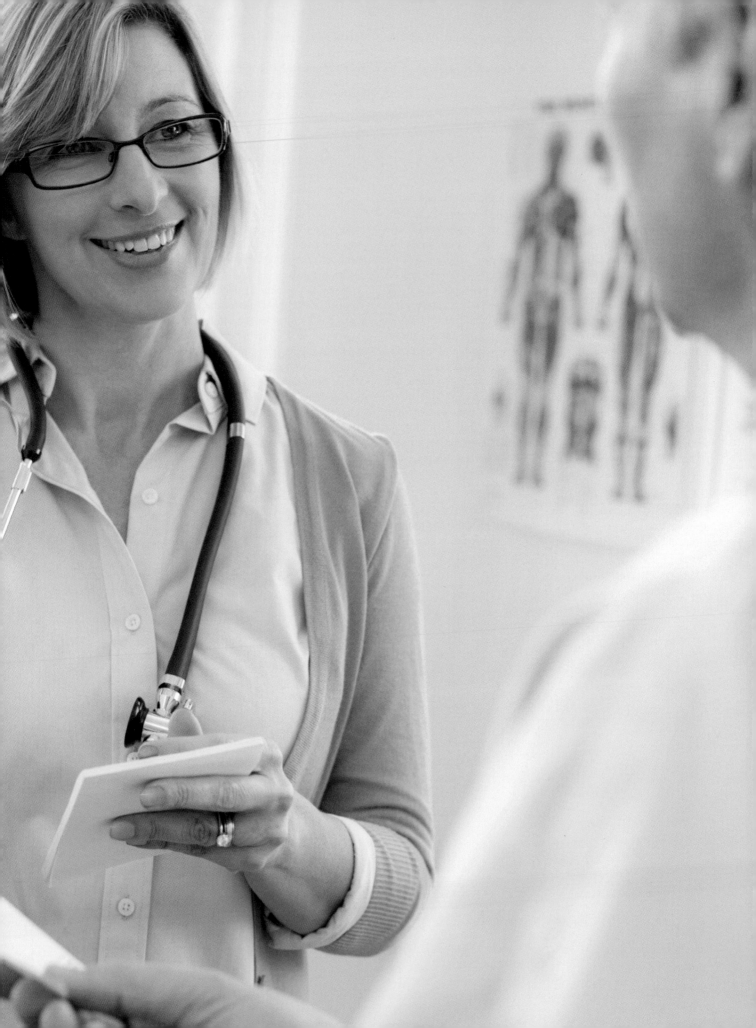

Cases

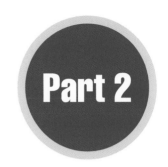

Part 2

Chapters

1   My baby is burning up   8
2   I need something for hay fever   10
3   I can't seem to shift this cough   12
4   My knee is very bad   14
5   I have migraine   16
6   I've come for my flu jab   18
7   He's a little terror   20
8   I've got a problem with my shoulder   22
9   I can't believe how much weight I've put on   24
10 It's my back passage   26
11 I am pregnant again   28
12 My baby has an upset tummy   30
13 My ear really hurts   32
14 I'm worried about my drinking   33
15 She cries all the time   34
16 I need something to help me sleep   36
17 My eye hurts   38
18 I think I should get this prostate test, doctor   40
19 I can't live with this pain much longer   41
20 I've got a red eye   44
21 I'm fed up with my spots   46
22 I've come for the results of my blood tests   48
23 I'd like to talk to you about HRT   50
24 I've got a bit of a discharge   52
25 I'm feeling tired and woozy   54
26 I think I need to get my blood pressure checked   56

27 Well, I'm pregnant   58
28 I've been feeling short of breath   60
29 She's coughing non-stop   62
30 I'm worried about my memory   64
31 I've got this pain in my chest, doctor   66
32 I've been having terrible stomach cramps   68
33 I'm concerned this mole has been growing   70
34 I seem to have lost weight   72
35 I'm worried about my erection   74
36 I think the cancer has got me   76
37 I'm all over the place these days   78
38 She's had tummy ache for two days   80
39 I don't want to have my period when I am on holiday   82
40 It's my leg   84
41 I'm having terrible diarrhoea   86
42 The nurse did my diabetes check last week. I'm here for the results   88
43 My skin is really itchy   90
44 Doctor, I'm just feeling really down   92
45 I've got a really bad burning in my stomach   93
46 I want to talk about my risk of breast cancer   94
47 I've got a terrible back ache   96
48 I'd like antibiotics please   98
49 I'm tired all the time   100
50 I'm worried about this lump, doctor   102

CASE

1 My baby is burning up

This afternoon Jay is brought in by his mother who tells you he's burning up. He's had a high fever since yesterday evening and wouldn't have any breakfast today. He only picked at his lunch. Jay seems reasonably happy sitting in his buggy.

What do you do now?

• Take a full **history of the current episode**.
• Has the **temperature** in fact been taken, and if so how (a forehead strip is inaccurate), and what was it? Have the parents **tried** giving him anything so far?
• Ask questions to establish **how ill** this child is: is he playing, socializing, smiling? Is he more drowsy than usual? Children with a fever may be a bit subdued but they should be alert. Is there evidence of dehydration? Ask the mother if his nappies have been drier than usual.
• Ask about **other symptoms such as cough, hoarse voice and rashes**. You already know his appetite is affected, so enquire about diarrhoea and vomiting.
• Establish his **immunization status**. This should be in the medical records (see Table 1.1).
• Ask about **contact** with anyone ill, and about foreign **travel**.

Ms Evans tells you that she didn't take the temperature, but she just knows Jay has a fever. Apart from being off his food, he vomited once after lunch, about two hours before coming to see you. He isn't coughing, and doesn't have hoarseness or diarrhoea. There may have been a rash last night, but Ms Evans thinks it is just Jay's eczema making a comeback. There has been no travel. Nobody at home has been unwell lately, but, ever since big sister Megan began playschool, both she and Jay have had a lot of snuffles.

Do you examine this child?

Yes. Many children dislike being examined, especially when they don't feel well, but don't rush or skimp. You need to check for red

URTI (usually viral)
Flu
Viral exanthems (e.g, chickenpox, rubella, measles)
Otitis media
Tonsillitis/scarlet fever
Chest infection
Septic arthritis
Meningitis/encephalitis
Sepsis (including streptococcal)
Toxic shock syndrome
Malaria
Other tropical diseases, e.g. Ebola
Kawasaki disease
Post-immunization
Dehydration
Factitious fever

Figure 1.1 Causes of fever.

flags that tell you this child may be seriously ill, and this includes taking the temperature.

You must also look for clues as to the cause of the fever. Remember that this may be the only chance to assess this child during his illness, and it must be done properly. The child will be more comfortable if you examine him on his mother's lap, and you don't undress him all at once: just get the mother to remove the clothes from his top half when you examine his chest, and the bottom half later in the examination.

> **Key point**
> Whenever you see a child, always ask yourself 'Is this child ill?'

List at least six important signs you should look for in determining how ill a child is.

The traffic light system can be useful for assessing febrile children (see Resources), but it is easier to remember red flags such as:

▶ Fever >38 °C in baby under 3 months or fever >39 °C in baby 3–6 months.
▶ Won't interact or socialize.
▶ Difficult to rouse.
▶ Pale or mottled skin.
▶ Dry mucous membranes.
▶ Reduced skin turgor.
▶ Capillary refill time greater than 3 seconds.
▶ Respiratory rate:
  • >60/min if under 6 months
  • >50/min if between 6 and 12 months
  • >40/min for children over 12 months.
▶ Indrawing of intercostal spaces.
▶ Grunting.
▶ Tachycardia:
  • >160/min if under 12 months
  • >150/min if 12–24 months old
  • >140/min if 2–5 years old.
▶ Non-blanching rash.
▶ Inability to move a limb.
▶ Bulging fontanelle.
▶ Focal neurological signs.
▶ High-pitched cry.
▶ Low oxygen sats

Can you now reassure the mother that it is only a virus?

No. Jay has a moderately high temperature, is off his food and you don't know what's wrong. The fact that you haven't found a focus of infection isn't necessarily reassuring. It could be a UTI, or the evolving stages of an illness, before any localizing signs appear. He may have one of the childhood exanthems, or septic arthritis or some other potentially serious infection.

> **Key point**
> Always remember that around half of all children with meningococcal disease aren't diagnosed at the first consultation.

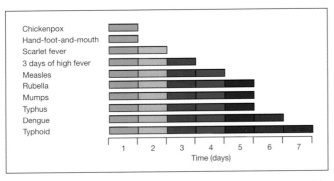

Figure 1.2 Usual prodromal phases of some infections, during which there may be fever and malaise.

What one test do you consider doing now?

Urine dipstick for WBCs, protein and nitrites.

Childhood UTIs

Most occur in the first year of life and present with vague symptoms such as fever (which can be recurrent) or vomiting, lethargy and poor feeding.

By the age of 11 years, 1% of boys and 4% of girls will have had a UTI.

▶ Over 30% of children with UTI have an underlying abnormality such as vesico-ureteric reflux, urethral valve or renal pathology. There is sometimes a family history.

Unfortunately Jay will not pass urine on demand. Your choice lies between giving the mother a bag to collect urine, or a sample pot and asking her to leave the child's nappy off until she has managed to collect a sample. Either way, you are unlikely to get a urine sample while he is still in the surgery.

Ms Evans looks at you expectantly. What do you advise her to do?

As there are no red flags (yet), it is reasonable to leave the urine sample till the morning. Meanwhile advise Ms Evans to keep Jay

Table 1.1 Chart of routine childhood immunizations.

When to immunize	Diseases protected against	Immunization site
Two months old	Diphtheria, tetanus, pertussis, polio and *Haemophilus influenzae* type b (Hib)	Thigh
	Pneumococcal disease	Thigh
	Rotavirus	By mouth
Three months old	Diphtheria, tetanus, pertussis, polio and Hib	Thigh
	Meningococcal group C disease (MenC)	Thigh
	Rotavirus	By mouth
Four months old	Diphtheria, tetanus, pertussis, polio and Hib	Thigh
	Pneumococcal disease	Thigh
Between 12 and 13 months old – within a month of the first birthday	Hib/Men C	Upper arm
	Pneumococcal disease	Upper arm
	Measles, mumps and rubella (German measles)	Upper arm
Two, three or four years old	Influenza	Usually nasal vaccine
Three years four months old or soon after	Diphtheria, tetanus, pertussis and polio	Upper arm
	Measles, mumps and rubella	Upper arm
Girls aged 12 to 13 years	Cervical cancer caused by HPV types 16 and 18 (and genital warts caused by 6 and 11)	Upper arm
Around 14 years old	Diphtheria, tetanus and polio	Upper arm
	MenC	Upper arm

cool by dressing him in lightweight clothes and giving him plenty of fluids. Tepid sponging is unhelpful and can be unpleasant.

If the temperature rises further or he seems uncomfortable, she could give paracetamol or ibuprofen in a formulation appropriate to his age, but fever is a normal physiological response to inflammation and it does not always need lowering.

It is wise to keep him away from other children, for example at nursery.

Give Ms Evans clear advice about when to return, and make sure she understands which symptoms are important. Include ▶ **drowsiness**, ▶ **clammy skin** and ▶ **rapid breathing**. Many parents fixate on the presence or absence of a ▶ **non-blanching rash** in meningitis/septicaemia and fail to realize that their child's general condition is at least as significant.

Tip

Remember that things change quickly with children. Safety-netting can save a young life, and could also save you from a serious complaint against you.

As it turns out, Jay's urine is normal the following morning. However his fever continues and he is irritable. When you see him two days later, he still has no focus of infection, and no red flags. Ms Evans has done some reading online and asks you if it is Kawasaki disease.

What are the main features of Kawasaki disease?

• High fever, often abrupt in onset, with irritability.
• Inflammation and irritation of the lips, mouth and/or tongue.
• Erythema, oedema and/or desquamation of the extremities.
• Bilateral dry conjunctivitis.
• Widespread non-vesicular rash.
• Cervical lymphadenopathy >1.5 cm in size.

To make the diagnosis, you would need fever and at least four of the other criteria. Kawasaki disease is rare but 80% of cases occur in the under-fives. It must be treated, usually as a paediatric or paediatric cardiology inpatient, to prevent complications such as coronary artery aneurysm.

Jay has none of the other features. He improves over the next couple of days without a precise diagnosis being made. When she comes to see you, you take the opportunity of mentioning routine immunizations.

Resources

NICE Feverish illness in children: Assessment and initial management in children younger than 5 years.

http://www.nice.org.uk/guidance/CG160

http://pathways.nice.org.uk/pathways/feverish-illness-in-children#content=view-node%3Anodes-use-the-traffic-light-system-to-assess-risk-of-serious-illness

NICE Urinary tract infection in children: Diagnosis, treatment and long-term management.

http://www.nice.org.uk/Guidance/CG54

Kawasaki disease Patient UK.

http://www.patient.co.uk/doctor/kawasaki-disease-pro

CASE

2 I need something for hay fever

Clare Davey, age 20 years
Student
PMH: constipation; anxiety; hay fever
Medication: lactulose

Clare Davey is a history student whose last two consultations were for constipation. Three months ago, one of your colleagues prescribed ispaghula husk. This did not help, so she returned to see another doctor. He noted she looked thin, and prescribed lactulose.

Today she wants something for hay fever that won't make her drowsy during exams. She has tried loratadine and cetirizine over the counter, but they do not help much, and she finds chlorphenamine too sedating. Her main symptoms are sneezing and runny nose. You therefore hope that a prescription of a steroid nasal spray will send her on her way, leaving you to catch up on lost time.

You ask briefly about her constipation and she says, 'I've got used to it.' You've never seen her before but you can't help noticing she looks thin, especially around the shoulders, even through a thick jumper. There is no record of her weight on the system.

What are your thoughts?

- She may be naturally slim.
- She may have an eating disorder, in which case it's your duty to assess her and initiate treatment.
- She may have lost weight unintentionally, which is your duty to investigate.

What three or four initial questions could you ask to sort out these three possibilities?

- 'How's your **general health**?'
- 'Has your **weight changed** over the last few months?'
- 'What are your **periods** like?' Amenorrhoea is common in anorexia nervosa, as well as bulimia even when the weight is normal.
- 'Do you feel the **cold**?' This isn't specific to eating disorders but can help distinguish hyperthyroidism (prefers the cold) from anorexia (often feels cold).

Clare says her general health is absolutely fine, but admits she's missed two periods. She can't possibly be pregnant, she adds, because she broke up with her boyfriend nearly a year ago and there's been nobody else. Her weight 'hasn't really changed'. She does feel the cold, but she just puts on extra layers. Today the sleeves of her jumper cover most of her hands.

You weigh her as this hasn't been done for quite a while according to the notes. She is 47 kg. At 5'6" (about 1.68 m) tall, her BMI is 16.6, low enough for anorexia nervosa (use centile charts for patients under 18).

You consider a pregnancy test in case what she's told you about timing is incorrect, but from Clare's weight and her responses so far you put an eating disorder at the top of your list.

Key point

According to NICE guidance on eating disorders, GPs should take the responsibility for the person's initial assessment and coordination of care.

Main types of eating disorders

- It's estimated that at least 6% of the population has an eating disorder.
- Eating disorders often start in the teens and are more common in women.
- But they can occur at almost any age, e.g. children as young as six years.
- Around a quarter are men.

Anorexia nervosa (about 0.6% population): low body weight due to preoccupation with weight and diet.

Bulimia nervosa (two to four times as common): episodes of binge eating and weight-loss behaviour (vomiting, fasting, excessive exercise). Weight is often normal.

Binge-eating disorder (the most common of all): recurrent persistent episodes of binge eating, at least three times a week, without compensatory weight loss behaviour. Weight may be normal or high.

The diagnosis of '**atypical eating disorder**' is sometimes still used when features don't fit any of the three main categories.

Of these eating disorders, anorexia seems the most likely diagnosis here.

What could you now ask to confirm this?

Your challenge is to tease out a fuller history, without losing your patient's trust, appearing judgmental, or antagonizing her. Remember she's likely to have already been interrogated or judged by her family and friends.

The **SCOFF questionnaire** can help in the diagnosis of eating disorders:

- Have you ever felt so uncomfortably full that you have had to make yourself **S**ick?
- Do you worry that you have ever lost **C**ontrol over what you eat?
- Have you gained or lost more than **O**ne stone over a three-month period?
- Do you believe yourself to be **F**at when others think you're thin?
- Would you say that **F**ood dominates your life?

A positive answer to two or more questions suggests anorexia or bulimia.

However, direct questioning such as this can be difficult so you may do better with a gentler start:

- 'Tell me **how things are** at the moment.' She might reveal sources of stress at home or at college.
- 'Tell me **about your weight**' and 'What would be your ideal weight?'
- 'Have you **dieted** or tried anything else to lose weight?' followed up by 'I realize that some people turn to various tablets...' Find out

if she eats with others (those with eating disorders often eat alone). Also ask about exercise and whether she goes to the gym.

• Ask about possible complications of eating disorders, e.g. dry skin, body hair, tiredness from anaemia, fainting spells, dental problems if vomiting.

• 'Tell me about your mood day-to-day.' This may reveal depression, or sources of stress, especially if you allow plenty of time for the answer.

• 'Have there been any illnesses in the family?' Sometimes there's a family history of mental illness, of anorexia or gross obesity.

Clare tells you that she has always felt fat and that her mother is very slim. She doesn't know what her ideal weight might be. She has tried laxatives but not diuretics or illicit drugs. She does not exercise regularly. All her time is taken up by her studies, and she wants to do well. She says she makes 'lots of healthy food' and eats mostly alone. She admits she may now have lost a bit too much weight. Her mood is 'fine' but she is worried about impending exams.

You now examine Clare. Apart from her weight, which you already checked, what are you looking for? Write down at least four things.

• **Pulse** and **BP**. There may be bradycardia or postural hypotension.
• **Temperature**. There can be hypothermia.
• **Circulation**. Acrocyanosis is common. Sometimes there's oedema, and in rare cases there can be gangrenous digits.
• Test **muscle power**. Doing a sit-up and getting up from a squatting position are both useful tests.

Her temperature, pulse and BP are normal. Her fingers are a bit cold. She can get up from a squatting position without using her arms, except to balance.

What do you do now?

The absence of physical findings does not mean you can ignore her eating disorder. First, you could discuss your concerns about her weight, then ask if she has considered this may be anorexia. This may enable you to get agreement that she'd benefit from help before things get out of hand.

Meanwhile, you want to do a few simple tests, if that's OK with her.

Clare readily agrees, mainly because, as she admits, she has less energy than she did, and can't study half the night as she used to.

What investigations do you consider?

• FBC, U&Es and creatinine. LFTs and albumin. Glucose.
• Consider an ECG, especially if BMI is under 15, or there is bradycardia.

All Clare's results come back normal. This is the case in most people with eating disorders. It's mildly reassuring, because it suggests her health is not currently at high risk.

CKS/NICE has a guide to determine who is most at risk. Low BMI, postural hypotension, bradycardia, poor muscle strength and abnormal blood tests are all significant. Some people need admission.

> **Tip**
> Remember anorexia nervosa is the most deadly of all mental health conditions.

Consider admission to hospital for any of the following

• Risk of suicide or severe self-harm (needs admission to acute psychiatry, not eating disorders unit).
• Home situation hinders recovery.
• Severe deterioration (may require admission to acute medical ward).
• Very low body weight (refer urgently if BMI <15).
• Medical complications (e.g. severe electrolyte disturbance, hypoglycaemia or severe intercurrent infection).
If considering *compulsory* admission (whatever your patient's age), get specialist advice. See Resources for details.

For everyone else, referral to the Community Mental Health Team (CMHT) or a specialist eating disorders unit is appropriate, depending on local provision.

Clare looks relieved when you suggest an eating disorders unit. But that doesn't mean success is within sight. It's worth making a further appointment to see her yourself, to keep an eye on her progress and to benefit from the rapport you have begun to build.

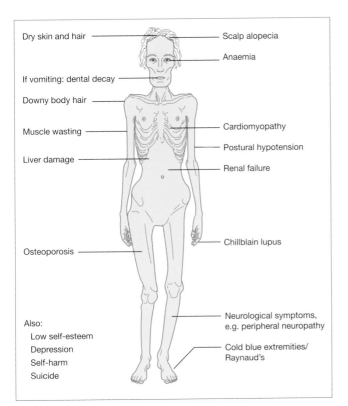

> **Tip**
> Be aware that a patient's weight sometimes appears to rise, if they drink a lot of water before their appointment or put heavy objects in their underclothes.

Resources

CKS/NICE Eating disorders.
  http://cks.nice.org.uk/eating-disorders#!scenario
BEAT the UK's leading eating disorders charity.
  http://www.b-eat.co.uk/

Figure 2.1 Complications of anorexia nervosa.

CASE

3

I can't seem to shift this cough

Peter Baker, age 61 years

Retired electrician and builder

PMH: hernia repair; repair to arm tendons after accident at work; mumps and measles as child; possible hypertension

Medication: nil

Mr Baker's cough started a few weeks ago, just after a trip to Spain where his son lives. He is not sure if he had a fever for a couple of days while he was away. Now he does not feel too well, and he wants an antibiotic.

The cough bothers him most at night. It is usually non-productive but there's some phlegm in the mornings. He never looks at the colour.

You see from the records that his blood pressure was high last year and he did not return to have it checked when he was advised to do so.

What do you need to know? Write down at least six questions to ask him now

- Does he **smoke**? This is a crucial question with suspected respiratory or cardiovascular symptoms.
- Has he coughed up **blood**? Haemoptysis occurs in infections, embolism and malignancy. Patients know it's sinister and don't always volunteer this symptom.
- Does he have **chest pain**?
- Has he lost weight? Ask also about other **systemic symptoms** such as fever, and enquire about 'any other symptoms' such as back pain.
- Have any of his family had a cough? Is there any **family history** of chest trouble? Think asthma, TB, other infections.
- Has there been other recent **travel**? Retired people often travel a lot. Was he well before he went away?
- Find out more about his work. Has he been exposed to **asbestos/** other potential hazards?

He used to smoke 30 a day but stopped about two years ago. A long while ago, he worked briefly with asbestos. There is no relevant FH, and no contact with pneumonia or TB. He feels a bit unwell but isn't sure if he has a fever. Nobody in his household is unwell. He thinks he was OK before they went to Spain, apart from a bit of a cough. Smoker's cough, he reckons, even though he had stopped smoking.

Cough in general practice

Most coughs are due to URTI but always consider other causes.

Acute cough (<3 weeks)
- URTI.
- Chest infection.
- Acute asthma; exacerbation of COPD.
- Thrombo-embolic disease (but most PEs are silent).
- Acute pneumothorax (especially in a young person).
- FB.

Cough between 3 and 8 weeks
- Post-infectious cough (common).
- Persistent infection.
- An early stage of a chronic cough.

Needs referral if there are any features to suggest lung cancer, TB or FB.

Chronic cough (>8 weeks)
- COPD (very common).
- Asthma.
- TB.
- Bronchiectasis.
- Lung cancer.
- FB aspiration.
- Interstitial lung disease, e.g. idiopathic pulmonary fibrosis.
- Hay fever, other forms of chronic rhinitis and post-nasal drip.
- GORD.
- Drug-induced, e.g. ACE inhibitors.

Not all need referral. **But refer urgently if there are features to suggest lung cancer, TB or FB.**

You ask to examine him. Write down five signs or checks you might look for, in addition to listening to his chest.

- Clubbing. As you do so, look for stained fingernails. Some smokers lie about giving up.
- Lymph nodes in the neck.
- PEFR.
- His weight may be useful if you have a previous value recorded.
- His BP, which was high last time. It's easy to focus on the patient's current symptom and forget outstanding tasks.

You find that he has lost 2 kg in weight in a month, though he tells you he tried to. BP is 164/98. No clubbing or stained fingers (often called 'nicotine stains', these are really due to tar). You think AE is reduced in the left lower lobe and there is some wheeze. No lymph nodes palpable in his neck. His PEFR is 410 (he is 6'1"). He coughs frequently during the examination and you notice the cough sounds a bit odd.

What is your differential diagnosis? Give at least four options.

- COPD.
- Carcinoma of the bronchus.
- Asbestosis.
- Chest infection.
- Asthma.

What do you do now?

Choose one or more of the following:
- reassure him
- tell him to get some cough syrup
- prescribe an antibiotic
- prescribe an inhaler
- get spirometry done
- request a CXR

General Practice Cases at a Glance, First Edition. Carol Cooper and Martin L Block. © 2017 John Wiley & Sons, Ltd. Published 2017 by John Wiley & Sons, Ltd.

- do a blood test
- bring him back for review, including blood pressure
- refer him urgently.

He should have a **CXR**, as he has lost weight and is at high risk of having lung cancer. An immediate chest **referral** under the two-week rule is also a good option especially if you can't get CXR result within a few days (see NICE guidelines in Resources). A **bronchodilator inhaler** would be reasonable. Cough syrups don't work, and there is no indication for an antibiotic. **Spirometry** is indicated as he almost certainly has COPD (the 'smoker's cough'). FBC, U&E, creatinine, lipids and glucose are reasonable from the hypertension angle, but unlikely to help you diagnose his cough. You have no basis for reassuring him, but you shouldn't alarm him unduly.

What do you tell him?

As with any cough for more than three weeks, this has to be taken seriously. You'll both know more after the x-ray. If he asks about the possibility of lung cancer, you must address this and let him know that it is on your list, but that doesn't mean he has it. Give him a follow-up appointment, and check that you have the right phone number for him in case you need to get in touch before then.

His chest x-ray report is faxed through the next day. It tells you he has hyper-inflated lungs as well as collapse at the left base. The mediastinum is wider than normal and his heart is enlarged.

The nurse has not yet done his spirometry. You refer him urgently to the chest physician.

Lung cancer

- Over 39 000 new cases a year in UK.
- Over 35 000 people die a year from lung cancer (more than breast and colorectal cancer combined).
- Now the main cause of cancer death in women.
- The UK's outcomes are worse than in the USA and many European countries, probably because of late referral and treatment. Treatment of advanced disease is usually disappointing, e.g. 12 weeks' chemotherapy only prolongs survival by eight weeks.
- At least 10% are not linked with smoking.
- At least 5% of lung cancers have a mutation in EGFR (epithelial growth factor receptor). New biologicals acting on EGFR can prolong survival in non-small-cell lung cancer, but not all UK centres in the UK test for it.

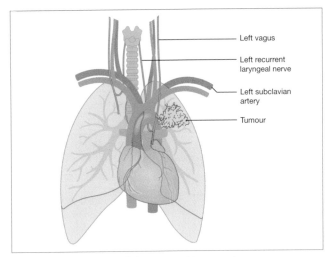

Figure 3.1 The course of the recurrent laryngeal nerves.

Ten days later, you hear that he has been diagnosed with cancer of his left lung as well as COPD. No wonder he had weight loss and an odd-sounding cough. The holiday was a red herring. Unfortunately Mr Baker is not a candidate for surgery as he has enlarged mediastinal nodes and recurrent laryngeal nerve involvement as well as COPD.

Recurrent laryngeal nerve palsy often presents with voice changes, but also causes a typically 'bovine' cough, caused by the expulsion of air past an open glottis. Remember that the course of the laryngeal nerve is not the same on both sides (Figure 3.1). The left recurrent laryngeal nerve extends down into the chest and loops under the arch of the aorta to return to the larynx. The right recurrent laryngeal nerve is shorter and loops around the subclavian artery. The left nerve is therefore more susceptible to disease than the right. While there are many possible causes of palsy, the most common are:

- bronchial carcinoma
- oesophageal carcinoma
- malignancy of the mediastinal lymph nodes.

The recurrent laryngeal nerves can also be affected by pathology in the neck (e.g. thyroid cancer or surgery).

Resources

CKS Cough.
    http://cks.nice.org.uk/cough#!topicsummary
NICE Lung cancer diagnosis and treatment.
    http://www.nice.org.uk/guidance/cg121

CASE
4
My knee is very bad

Giovanna Harris, age 67 years
Housewife and carer
PMH: mild asthma; hysterectomy; operation for bunions; postnatal depression
Medication: beclomethasone and salbutamol inhalers

Mrs Giovanna Harris has had a painful right knee for 'quite some time' but it has been much worse in the last eight or nine months. It is especially bad going downstairs. But sometimes she just sits on the sofa in the evening and it's so painful that she doesn't know what to do. She has already tried cod liver oil and tablets from the health shop which were no good at all.

What could you ask now? Write down 10 or more useful questions.

• 'Tell me **more about the pain**.' Is it the front or back of the knee? Clarify what makes it better, if anything, and its other characteristics.
• 'Have you **injured** your knee?' Recent or long past trauma are both significant.
• 'Is it bad **at night?**' ► Pain mostly or solely at night can suggest tumour.
• 'Do you get **swelling**?' This could be effusion or synovitis.
• 'Does the knee **feel stiff**?' Morning stiffness for >30 minutes suggests inflammation.
• 'Does it ever give way?' This could be due to ligamentous laxity, or to quads wasting.
• 'Does it lock, so that you can't straighten it completely?' Locking suggests a loose body or a meniscus injury.
• 'How are your **other joints**?' It might be part of a more widespread arthropathy.
• 'Do you **feel well** in yourself?' ► Systemic symptoms occur in inflammatory arthritis, and with sepsis. Always take weight loss seriously.
• 'Do you have any **skin problems**?' Psoriatic arthropathy can be limited to one knee.
• 'Does anyone in your family have joint trouble?'
• 'How much does it bother you on a day-to-day basis?' Find out what, if anything, it stops her doing. Asking her to **score her pain** on a scale of nought to 10 can be useful too.
• Remember to ask her what she thinks it might be, and what she hopes you might do for her. These open questions can unlock your patient's **ICE**.

Mrs Harris says there was a knee injury many years ago while ice-skating when she first came to the UK. It was swollen and treated with bandages. Her knee is only a little stiff in the mornings. It hasn't swollen lately and doesn't lock, but it feels 'a bit wobbly' sometimes. When she is walking, the bones feel like they're rubbing together. The pain is mostly at the front of the knee and there is not much pain at night. She can't run or dance, and doesn't do any sports anyway as she is very busy looking after her mother who is 92 and 'has lost her mind'. She is the only carer.

Her general health is good, and there is no other joint problem. Nobody in her family seems to have arthritis or anything like that, though her mother's hands are very knobbly. She isn't sure what you might do for her, but she doesn't want surgery.

You decide to examine Mrs Harris. What do you check in particular? Write down six things.

• You may already have noticed her general appearance including **gait**. If not, observe how she walks.
• The hands may show **Heberden's nodes**, typical of osteoarthritis.
• Turning to the knees, is there **wasting** of her right knee? Look also for **swelling** and ► **redness**.
• Is the knee in varus or valgus? Either suggests OA.
• Check for **tenderness**. The site can be helpful (e.g. joint line tenderness in meniscal injury).
• Check the **range of movement** (ROM), and whether movement hurts.
• Test for ligamentous laxity: the collateral ligaments are easier to check than the cruciates.
• Assess her for generalized joint **hypermobility**. If you don't test for it, this can get overlooked.
• Examine the **hip**. Knee pain can be referred from the hip, though this is more common in children.

On examination, Mrs Harris is overweight. She weighs 73 kg and measures 1.6 m so her BMI is 28.5. She walks well. There are Heberden's nodes (Figure 4.1). Her right knee is not swollen or red, but the quads are wasted. She is tender on either side of the patella. ROM is good. There is patello–femoral crepitus which you consider to be irrelevant. You find no ligamentous laxity or any signs of hypermobility. She does not have psoriasis. The left knee and both hips are normal.

Some causes of knee pain

Younger patients (age 16–50)
• Injuries (e.g. fracture, ligamentous tear).
• Meniscus tear.
• Osgood–Schlatter's disease.
• Osteochondritis dissecans.
• Inflammatory arthritis.
• ► Septic arthritis.
• ► Osteomyelitis.
• Joint hypermobility.
• Patello–femoral tracking problem.
• Early OA following trauma.
• Bursitis.

Older patients (over 50)
• Injuries (e.g. fracture, ligamentous tear).
• Meniscus degeneration.
• OA.
• Inflammatory arthritis.
• ► Septic arthritis.
• ► Osteomyelitis.
• Patello–femoral tracking problem.
• Bursitis.
• Gout or pseudogout.
• Baker's cyst.

General Practice Cases at a Glance, First Edition. Carol Cooper and Martin L Block. © 2017 John Wiley & Sons, Ltd. Published 2017 by John Wiley & Sons, Ltd.

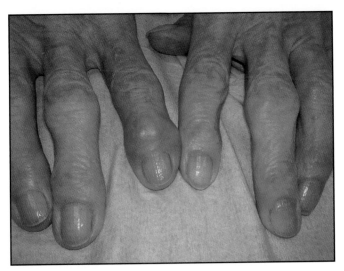

Figure 4.1 Heberden's nodes.

Source: Drahreg01 https://commons.m.wikimedia.org/wiki/File:Heberden-Arthrose.JPG. Used under CCA 3.0.

What are your thoughts now? Write down at least two possibilities.

- Osteoarthritis or degenerative joint disease (DJD).
- Late consequence of a previous meniscus tear.
- It could still be an inflammatory disorder but this is much less likely.

Does she need a scan or an x-ray?

No. MRI scanning is the gold-standard test, but it would be impossible to scan every painful knee presenting to the GP, and it is unlikely to help in management here.

An x-ray might show a narrowed joint space, osteophytes and/or subchondral changes, but around 70% of people with knee pain have changes of OA on x-ray, and these correlate poorly with symptoms.

You have a working diagnosis of OA knee. What are your management options?

Lifestyle measures are the most important, especially building up quads and losing weight (if appropriate). Regular exercise like walking can be beneficial, with the right footwear.

In terms of **analgesia**, paracetamol can be worth trying, though it may not be very effective. Topical NSAIDs can help. Oral NSAIDs with PPI cover are worth trying next. A paracetamol and opioid combination (e.g. co-dydramol) is the next step after that. Topical capsaicin is an option too.

Physiotherapy has an important role, and from there the next step up would be **specialist assessment**, which may lead to joint injection, arthroscopy or joint replacement. Severe symptomatic OA knee merits **knee replacement**. The Oxford Knee Score can help in assessment.

Mrs Harris has already tried paracetamol and was disappointed. You decide NSAIDs would be unwise as aspirin and ibuprofen have given her asthma attacks in the past, and you settle on co-codamol which she is happy to try. You give her a leaflet on quads exercise and ask the **physio** to give her one-off advice, which may include modifying her activities to protect her knee.

Mrs Harris is aware that she needs to lose weight. You also suggest that she get some help in looking after her mother (who is a patient with another practice), and she might like to join a carers' group for ideas and support. You're pleased to find that she agrees with your suggestions.

Resources

CKS/NICE Knee pain – assessment.
   http://cks.nice.org.uk/knee-pain-assessment#!scenario

Oxford knee score.
   www.orthopaedicscore.com/scorepages/oxford_knee_score.html

Arthritis Research UK (charity with range of publications for patients and health professionals, including exercise sheets).
   www.arthritisresearchuk.org/

CASE

5 I have migraine

> **Amy Liu, age 19 years**
> Student
> PMH: nil
> Medication: antihistamines for hay fever

Amy is a university student, originally from Hong Kong. She has had bad headaches on and off for about three months, and she thinks it's migraine. She is slim and does not smoke, and she rarely drinks alcohol.

What should you ask in trying to establish whether this is migraine? Write down at least six questions.

- Ask about **laterality.** Migraine is classically one-sided (the word comes from 'hemicrania'), but exceptions occur.
- Is it associated with **nausea** or **vomiting**? These point to migraine, but aren't exclusive to it.
- 'Are you more sensitive to **light** or **sound**?' This is typical of migraine, but meningitis also causes dislike of bright lights.
- 'Are you still **able to function**?' Many migraine sufferers cannot carry on with work or their usual activities because it worsens the headache.
- 'Is your **vision** affected?' Visual aura occurs in about 15% of migraines. There can be other focal symptoms too.
- Ask about **family history**. There's typically a genetic element.

Tip
Many people use the word 'migraine' to mean a really bad headache. Other patients, especially those with a family history, understand a bit more about it.

Amy's headaches are frontal and bilateral. They're worse in the evening, and not associated with aura or any other symptoms. Sometimes they last a day or two. She usually manages to soldier on with her studying, although less effectively as usual. She isn't sure about her family history, but offers to ring her mum in Hong Kong to ask her. You tell Amy that's not necessary at this point.

What are some important causes of headache? Write down at least 10, in roughly descending order of seriousness.

- Head trauma with fracture and/or intracranial bleed.
- Other forms of cerebral haemorrhage (e.g. subarachnoid).
- Encephalitis or meningitis.
- Space-occupying lesion.
- Carbon monoxide poisoning.
- Giant cell arteritis (especially in over-50s).
- Acute glaucoma.
- Migraine.
- Cluster headache.
- Tension-type headache.
- Trigeminal neuralgia.
- Other types of referred pain (e.g. from neck, teeth, jaw, sinuses).
- Depression.

- Fever (e.g. flu).
- Medication over-use headache (also called 'chronic daily headache').
- Medication side effect (e.g. vasodilators, SSRIs).
- Illicit drugs.
- Hangover.

Most headaches are not sinister. In general practice, 90% are **primary headaches**, according to the classification of the International Headache Society. These include **tension-type headache**, **migraine**, **cluster headache** and **other primary headaches** (e.g. benign sexual headache). Of these, tension-type and migraine are the most common, and they may be complicated by **analgesic over-use**.

However, that does not stop patients occasionally having serious conditions that must not be missed.

With this in mind, what are some useful questions you could ask to help diagnose Amy's headache?

- ► 'Have you hit your head recently?' Any history of **head trauma** in the last three months or so is important.
- 'How did your headache start?' ► **Sudden onset** (like being hit with a cricket or baseball bat) is typical of SAH, but some evolve a bit more slowly. Cough or exercise can also provoke SAH.
- 'Do you have a **fever**?' Consider meningitis or encephalitis, alongside more common causes.
- ► 'Have you **felt sick or been sick**?' Effortless vomiting without nausea is a hallmark of raised intracranial pressure, though nausea and vomiting occur in migraine.

Tip
Ensure the patient understands what you mean here. To Americans, for example, 'being sick' does not mean vomiting. It means being unwell.

- ► 'Do you have **other symptoms**?' Seizures are sinister, while weakness, or other focal neurological symptoms, can suggest migraine or something more serious. Visual symptoms occur in migraine as well as acute narrow-angle glaucoma.
- 'Is your **neck** stiff or painful?' Neck stiffness can occur in meningitis, though it can also be a clue to referred pain, e.g. from whiplash injury.
- 'Do you often take **tablets for your headache**?' Analgesic overuse headache is the most common cause of secondary headache. Amy's answers are reassuring. She has had no head injuries, no fever and certainly no fits or other symptoms. Each headache usually begins gradually towards the end of the day. There's no nausea or vomiting. She has only tried painkillers 'a couple of times', and says neither paracetamol nor ibuprofen helped. Her neck and back are 'OK'.

What further questions might you ask? Write down three.

- Ask about low mood and other symptoms of **depression**.
- Ask about **stress**.
- Ask about visual problems and her most recent **eye check**.
- Inquire about her use of **computers**, and any **leisure** activities (e.g. rowing, weight-lifting, playing a wind instrument which might lead to jaw or neck problems).

General Practice Cases at a Glance, First Edition. Carol Cooper and Martin L Block. © 2017 John Wiley & Sons, Ltd. Published 2017 by John Wiley & Sons, Ltd.

Amy has no symptoms of depression. She is 'quite stressed' doing her course in chemistry, but she loves it. Although she has no family here, she has made lots of friends. Her eyesight is fine. She wears glasses and last saw the optician about eight months ago. She uses the computer a lot, especially during the week. Occasionally she goes to the gym, mainly to swim.

Do you examine Amy?

Yes, you should. While a serious cause for her headaches is unlikely, you haven't ruled out all the possibilities. You might also gain useful clues as to the cause. Finally, examination can be reassuring to the patient and indicates you're taking the symptoms seriously.

What in particular will you examine? Write down three things.

- BP.
- Neck.
- Neurological examination.
- In over-50s, check for ▶ tenderness over the temporal arteries.

Tip

When short of time for a CNS examination, concentrate on the motor side rather than the sensory.

In this case, you should check the fundi for papilloedema and test most of the cranial nerves (e.g. III, IV, VI, VII and XII).

Check power in the limbs and the plantar reflexes. Also test coordination and balance (e.g. finger–nose test and heel–toe walking).

Amy's BP is 116/76. Her optic discs, cranial nerves, power, heel–toe walking and finger–nose test are all normal. Plantars are down-going. Her neck has FROM, but her trapezius muscles are a bit tender.

What do you think?

There is no sign of anything sinister, and this sounds like tension headache and/or referred pain from the neck.

Amy then tells you she mainly uses a laptop, 'like every student'. This is significant because the screen can't be at the right height for vision and the keys at the right height for the upper limb, unless there's an external monitor or keyboard. It may explain the timing of her headaches. Amy goes away and says she will get an external keyboard. You give her advice about taking regular breaks away from the screen, and suggest she returns to see you if her headaches persist.

Six weeks later, she phones you at 2 pm with sudden-onset headache while at the gym. She managed to get back to her flat but this is the worst headache ever and she feels terrible, with nausea.

What do you do now?

(a) Visit her right away?
(b) Visit later if she doesn't improve?
(c) Send her to hospital by ambulance?
(d) Give her an appointment for later in the week?

You must take this seriously so (a) and (c) are the best options. Patients with a benign cause for their symptoms can develop more acute and more sinister conditions too.

You double-check her address, make sure there's somebody with her and call an ambulance for her.

Several days later, you learn that she was diagnosed with SAH due to ruptured berry aneurysm, and is now doing well. Via Amy's parents, the neurosurgery registrar found out there was a family history of berry aneurysm.

SAH is unrelated to her original headaches, and nobody could fault your original assessment and management. You can't help wondering, however, whether the haemorrhage might have been avoided if Amy had phoned her mother to obtain a family history.

Berry aneurysms

About 80% of SAHs are due to ruptured berry aneurysms.
About 1 in every 25 adults has one or more berry aneurysms.
Family history can increase the risk of developing berry aneurysms. There is also a link with autosomal dominant polycystic disease.

Factors increasing risk of rupture:
- size of aneurysm >7 mm
- high BP
- drug use (e.g. cocaine)
- smoking
- excess alcohol.

Resources

CKS: Headache assessment.
  http://cks.nice.org.uk/headache-assessment#!topicsummary
SIGN (Scottish Intercollegiate Guidelines Network): Diagnosis and management of headache in adults.
  http://www.sign.ac.uk/pdf/qrg107.pdf

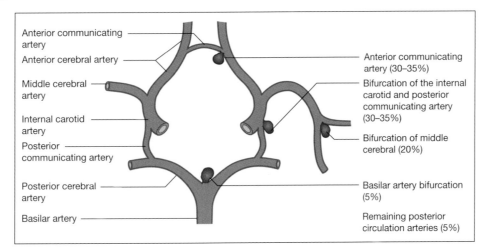

Figure 5.1 Location of berry aneurysms.

CASE

6 I've come for my flu jab

> **Mrs Millie Brown, age 81 years**
> Retired
> PMH: hypertension; high cholesterol; ex-smoker (gave up 20 years ago)
> Medication: amlodipine 5 mg od, ramipril 5 mg daily, atorvastatin 20 mg od

Mrs Brown comes to see you to get her blood pressure checked and her flu jab. She has just returned from spending a few days with her family in Devon. She is a widow and lives alone.

Before checking her BP, you check her pulse and you note that she is in an irregularly irregular rhythm. She has no history of arrhythmia and no other history of cardiac problems. Mrs Brown tells you she feels fine and not to worry.

You speak to the practice nurse who agrees to do an ECG on Mrs Brown after her next patient.

Mrs Brown returns 20 minutes later with an ECG (Figure 6.1).

What is the diagnosis?

Atrial fibrillation.

What questions would you like to ask Mrs Brown now?

You should enquire about any **symptoms**.

- How does she feel?
- Any breathlessness or chest pain?
- Any dizziness?
- Any unusual recent symptoms (e.g. to suggest a recent stroke or TIA)?

You should enquire about **possible triggers**.

- Has she been unwell recently?
- What is her alcohol intake?

Mrs Brown tells you that she feels pretty much fine, certainly no chest pain. One thing she has been noticing over the past few months is that she does get more breathless than she used to. When she walks to the shops, she has to stop two or three times to catch her breath. This has been over the past few months. She had put this down to getting old, and hadn't thought it worthy of troubling the doctor.

She hasn't noticed any unusual symptoms recently, definitely nothing to suggest a stroke or TIA. She only drinks on special occasions. Just a little glass of sherry.

Can you name at least five potential causes of AF?

- Hypertension.
- Ischaemic heart disease.
- Valvular heart disease (e.g. mitral valve disease).
- Heart failure.
- Infections (e.g. chest infection).
- PE.
- Lung cancer.
- Thyrotoxicosis.
- Diabetes.
- Electrolyte disturbance.
- Alcohol excess.

What examination would you like to do?

You should examine Mrs Brown's cardiovascular system and also her respiratory system. She is complaining of breathlessness. This could be due to her AF, or she could have a respiratory cause of AF.

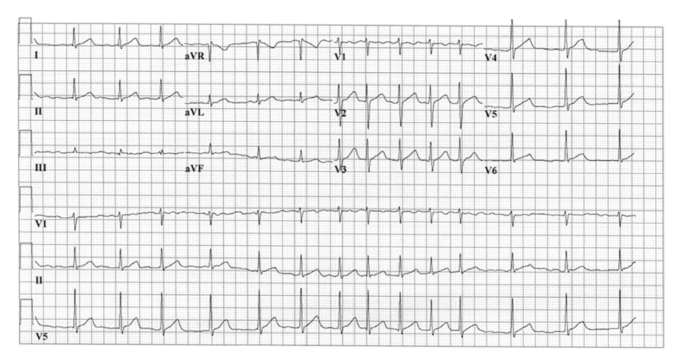

Figure 6.1 Mrs Brown's ECG.

Source: CardioNetworks https://commons.wikimedia.org/wiki/File:Afib_ecg_(CardioNetworks_ECGpedia).jpg. Used under CCA 3.0.

General Practice Cases at a Glance, First Edition. Carol Cooper and Martin L Block. © 2017 John Wiley & Sons, Ltd. Published 2017 by John Wiley & Sons, Ltd.

Examination findings

- chest clear
- CVS
  - heart rhythm – irregularly irregular, rate 98
  - soft systolic murmur (grade I), loudest at the apex with no radiation
  - BP (manual) 116/78
  - no ankle oedema.

How would you explain the diagnosis of AF to Mrs Brown?

It's best to keep your explanation clear, avoiding medical jargon. Try it out. How about something like this: 'Mrs Brown, you have a condition called atrial fibrillation. This is where your heart beats irregularly and often quite fast. We take it seriously because it can make you feel unwell and it can increase your risk of getting other conditions like stroke.'

Do you need to admit Mrs Brown to hospital now?

No. She does not have any features that require her to be admitted.

> **AF – when to refer**
>
> Admit (or refer), if the person has AF and:
> - pulse >140 or systolic BP <90
> - is **unwell**, e.g. loss of consciousness, severe dizziness, ongoing chest pain or increasing breathlessness
> - has **complications** of AF, e.g. stroke, TIA or acute heart failure.

What tests should you arrange for Mrs Brown?

All patients with AF should get:
- **ECG** (already done)
- **blood tests**: U+E, TFTs, glucose/Hba1c, calcium, lipids.

Also consider whether or not to do a **chest x-ray** and/or **echocardiogram**.

Does Mrs Brown need a CXR?

Yes – she has breathlessness and she is an ex-smoker. You need to exclude lung cancer, a potential cause of AF.

Does she need an echo?

Again yes. She has AF in the presence of a murmur, so it is worth assessing her for valvular disease.

What are the important areas you need to cover in your management?

1 Treat any underlying cause.
2 Control rate.
3 Consider rhythm control (i.e. cardioversion).
4 Consider need for anticoagulation.

Treat any underlying cause

You are waiting for the results of your tests above, but nothing has come up yet.

Control rate

- **Betablocker**, e.g. bisoprolol (unless asthmatic).
- Rate-limiting **calcium-channel blocker**, e.g. diltiazem or verapamil (unless heart failure).

Table 6.1 CHA2DS2VASc.

		SCORE
C	Congestive heart failure (or left ventricular systolic dysfunction)	1
H	Hypertension	1
A2	Age ≥75 years	2
D	Diabetes mellitus	1
S2	Stroke or TIA	2
V	Vascular disease (e.g. IHD, peripheral artery disease)	1
A	Age 65–74 years	1
Sc	Sex	1

A score of 0 is low risk and may not require anticoagulation
A score of 1 is 'low moderate', consider anticoagulation (e.g. warfarin or rivaroxaban)
A score of 2 or above is 'moderate–high' – anticoagulation advised

You start her on a low dose of betablocker for rate control, bisoprolol 1.25 mg daily.

Cardioversion

Refer to a cardiologist for consideration of rhythm-control treatment (cardioversion), in addition to prescribing a rate-control treatment, if the person has:
- AF with a reversible cause (for example a chest infection)
- heart failure thought to be primarily caused, or worsened, by AF
- new-onset AF.

On discussion with Mrs Brown you decide against cardioversion.

Consider need for anticoagulation

Do you know of any tools used for this?

There are a few tools used, e.g. CHADS and also the CHA2DS-2VASC.

Using Table 6.1, calculate Mrs Brown's score.

She scores 4. You refer her to the anticoagulation clinic for consideration of warfarin.

When should you follow her up?

In Mrs Brown's case as she is only mildly symptomatic and her rate is not excessively high, it would be good to follow her up in two weeks to assess response to rate control (you may have to up-titrate the betablocker) and review her results.

What must you not forget to do before she goes?

Give her a flu jab.

Postscript

Sadly Mrs Brown's CXR did show a likely malignancy. You referred her under the two-week rule and a diagnosis of carcinoma of the lung was made.

Resources

CKS NICE Atrial Fibrillation.
   http://cks.nice.org.uk/atrial-fibrillation

CASE

7 He's a little terror

Kai Johnson, age 5 years
PMH: nil of note
Medication: nil

Five-year old Kai bounces into the consulting room ahead of his mother Imelda Ryan who says, 'I can't control him. I'm sure there's something wrong.' Kai is the middle of Imelda's three children, and very unlike his older brother Luke or his little sister Katrina. He's constantly on the go and she's worn out. His mood changes a lot and he's prone to outbursts 'like toddler tantrums'. While Imelda tells you this, Kai is busy taking books off your shelf.

What important points should your history cover? Write down at least six.

There are two main areas to cover: details of the problem, and how the mother/family manages.
• Take a **full history of the problem** and when it began. Does the challenging behaviour occur only at home, or only with one or two specific people?
• Ask about the **past medical history**, including the birth, and Kai's **development**.
• Ask about **possible triggers**: a new baby, house move, change in partner, family crisis or illness, bullying at school.
• What is his **concentration** like? Many young children have trouble staying 'on task'. If a child can pay attention at home but not at school, or vice versa, it's not ADHD.
• Inquire about **other symptoms** too, e.g. disturbed sleep, eating problems, toileting issues. You'd expect a five-year old to be clean and dry by day, but 20% still wet the bed, and this can cause huge frustration for parent and child.
• Who is in the **household** and what do they do? Don't make assumptions about Imelda: many women with three children go out to work.
• **How does the mother manage** Kai? Is anyone else involved, and are they supportive of her? You're looking for conflict or inconsistency between the adults who care for him, and any hints of violence towards Kai. Does anyone in the family have health problems (e.g. depression), or abuse alcohol or drugs? ► Always remember the possibility of child abuse.
Imelda tells you it's tough because Kai has always been a handful. He eats OK but has 'never slept a whole night in his life'. Kai's concentration is bad. He started school recently and he's disruptive there too, with occasional aggression towards classmates. Her current boyfriend (not Kai's father) finds it difficult too, and sometimes drinks too much, but 'he's a good man, he wouldn't lay a finger on him'. He works as a mechanic and doesn't do drugs, though Kai's dad did 'quite a lot of coke'. They are no longer in contact. Imelda feels guilty about having used cocaine herself a couple of times when pregnant with Kai, but the pregnancy and birth were normal.

There haven't been any changes since the boyfriend moved in nearly two years ago when their baby arrived. Imelda is a stay-at-home mum and tries to provide a normal family life but doesn't get any support from her parents. They live nearby, but were horrified when she first got pregnant at 17 by 'a black man' and they haven't had much to do with her since. Imelda left school without completing her A-levels.

As she tells you all this, Kai is busy dismantling the paper roll on your examination couch, and ignores his mother's warning to stop it. He stops momentarily when you tell him to, and you manage to have a brief exchange. He smiles cheekily and makes eye contact as he replies to your questions: his name is Kai, he is five years old and he likes football.

What are your thoughts now?

Kai's behaviour could be due to **domestic circumstances**.

However from the history and what you see of Kai, **ADHD** is a possibility. He is impulsive and hyperactive. This appears persistent and occurs in different settings (home, school, GP surgery). But **autistic spectrum disorder** is also a plausible diagnosis. Although these two neurodevelopmental disorders are distinct they can both lead to challenging behaviour.

Attention deficit hyperactivity disorder (ADHD)

There is no diagnostic test for ADHD, so the history is crucial. Establish exactly what the parent means and whether they have realistic expectations of how children of that age should behave.
  Children with ADHD can show:
• **hyperactivity and impulsive behaviour**
• **inattention.**
They do not need to have both features. Children with inattention (attention deficit disorder or ADD) are often diagnosed later because symptoms are less obvious. The features must occur in more than one situation (e.g. home and school) and be out of keeping with the child's age.
Hyperactive/impulsive behaviour
• fidgeting
• inability to sit still
• unable to wait their turn
• doing things without thinking
• inappropriate behaviour
• talking a lot
• not sleeping much.
Inattention often means
• having a short attention span, even for enjoyable things
• being easily distracted
• leaving tasks unfinished
• losing or forgetting things
• appearing disorganized
• being unable to follow instructions
• being difficult to control in class and at home.
As a result, the child may feel frustrated and have mood swings, outbursts of aggression and even low self-esteem and depression.
  ADHD is usually obvious before the age of 6, and persists into adolescence and even adulthood. By 25, about 15% of those diagnosed in childhood still have symptoms.
  ADHD can co-exist with other problems.
  Diagnosis should be made by a specialist in secondary care.
Management
• advising parents/carer about coping with behaviour, e.g. establishing boundaries, being consistent, showing love without indulging the child

---

- structured daily routine
- possibly drug treatment (e.g. methylphenidate, atomoxetine), especially for inattention – this is prescribed in secondary care
- support groups such as ADDISS and CHADD.

Autism and autistic spectrum disorder

Autistic spectrum disorder (ASD) refers to a group of disorders under the general heading of the **pervasive developmental disorders** (PDD). Their common characteristic is disordered social interaction and communication.

The term includes **autism**, **Asperger syndrome** (intellect in normal range; no significant language delay), pervasive developmental disorder not otherwise specified (PDD-NOS) and childhood disintegrative disorder. Together these affect around 1% or more of the population, depending on criteria used for diagnosis.

Intellectual ability ranges from severely learning disabled up to normal or even superior intellect. **Language skills** range from muteness right up to excellent speech.

There are three hallmarks of autism.
- **Impaired social interaction:** the child is aloof and uninterested in people, or socially clumsy and finds it hard to initiate interactions.
- **Impaired communication:** speech may be abnormal in intonation and the child also has difficulty with non-verbal communication.
- **Impaired social imagination:** difficulty with pretend play, and even with appreciating that others have a different point of view.

In addition there may be the following.
- Repetitive or stereotyped behaviour: lining up objects, flapping their arms, collecting things, learning a narrow range of facts obsessively.
- Lack of joint attention behaviour: typically young children point out things to others, and observe their gaze to see what they're watching but those with autism may not.
- Hyperactivity, lack of cooperation and difficult behaviour.

Diagnosis can be difficult. There's no good screening test but any red flags should lead to a full assessment:

- ▶ no babbling by 12 months
- ▶ no gesturing (pointing, waving, saying bye-bye) by 12 months
- ▶ no response to own name by 12 months
- ▶ no single words by 16 months
- ▶ no spontaneous two-word phrases by 24 months
- ▶ prefers playing alone
- ▶ unusual attachment to objects (usually but not always a toy)
- ▶ any loss of language or social skills at any age.

Whatever the cause of Kai's behaviour, it's clear that the mother is **stressed** and **needs support** in coping.

Are there any other questions it might be useful to ask now?

- The **family history**. Both autism and ADHD can run in families, but with ADHD there's sometimes a useful clue if one of the parents (usually the father) was exactly the same as a child. Ask about Imelda and her siblings as well as Kai's father.

- You could also ask Imelda **what she thinks the problem is**. Most parents have a hunch. It may be right, or it may be wrong, but it is worth eliciting ideas, concerns and expectations, as it can help you find a mutually satisfactory way forward.

Imelda asks you if the problems are down to MMR vaccine, or something he eats, or else the coke she took in pregnancy.

What do you tell her?

You haven't made a diagnosis yet, but you can be fairly certain that both MMR and foods are blameless here, so it's reasonable to reassure her on that score. Cocaine is absorbed more quickly in pregnancy and it can have a number of adverse effects, but there's no evidence that one or two uses of the drug will lead to long-term problems.

Cocaine in pregnancy

Drug use often goes hand in hand with other risk factors, so it is hard to be dogmatic about its effects. The evidence suggests that cocaine use in pregnancy is linked with adverse effects on the fetus including:
- miscarriage
- placental abruption
- premature labour
- stillbirth
- poor growth in the womb
- abnormal CNS development
- neonatal withdrawal symptoms
- poor sleeping
- poor feeding.

Poor growth in childhood and learning difficulties are also potential risks.

As in non-pregnant women, cocaine can raise pulse and BP, and cause arrhythmias.

What do you do now?

- A **paediatric opinion** is in order. You could refer Kai to the community paediatrician or a hospital-based specialist. Alternatively, you could review Kai in a few weeks and try to make a fuller assessment, but this is unlikely to help much.
- **Social worker** involvement is desirable here. Some social workers also have expertise with ADHD families.
- You could speak to the **health visitor** about the family's needs in general. The health visitor may have seen Kai as well as the younger sibling recently.
- You should arrange to see Kai and his mother again. Families in difficulty can slip through the system and it is often the GP who provides continuity.

Resources

CKS/NICE Attention deficit hyperactivity disorder.
    http://cks.nice.org.uk/attention-deficit-hyperactivity-disorder
CKS/NICE Autism in children.
    http://cks.nice.org.uk/autism-in-children
National Autistic Society.
    www.autism.org.uk/
Cressman AM, Natekar A, Kim E, Koren G, Bozzo P. Cocaine abuse during pregnancy. J Obstet Gynaecol Can 2014; 36(7): 628–631.
    www.jogc.ca/abstracts/full/201407_DrugsinPregnancy_1.pdf
Southampton University Hospitals NHS Trust patient information sheet: Cocaine and Pregnancy.
    www.uhs.nhs.uk/Media/Controlleddocuments/
    Patientinformation/Pregnancyandbirth/
    Cocaineandpregnancy-patientinformation.pdf

CASE

8

I've got a problem with my shoulder

Home visit

Mavis Baker, age 81 years

Widow

PMH: OA – bilateral hip and knee: left knee replacement five years ago, right knee replacement two years ago

Medication: nil

Housebound; lives in a bungalow with daughter June who is her carer

---

Mrs Baker has asked for a visit as she is having shoulder pain for the last two weeks. She thinks she may have pulled a muscle but as it is not getting better she wonders if this could be arthritis beginning. You put her down for a home visit. She tells you she is on her own as daughter June is out at work. She tells you she may take some time to get to the door, so asks you to be patient with her.

You arrive and ring the bell, Mrs Baker can be heard slowly making her way over to the front door. She opens the door with one hand on her Zimmer frame. She leads you into the front room and you both sit down.

When does your consultation begin?

Before the consultation has formally begun, you have had the opportunity to start to gather some useful information. Think about what you have learned already about Mrs Baker. Her mobility is poor and, as she uses a Zimmer, her shoulder strength is important. The state of her home may also give you some useful information. As you walk with your patient down the corridor, always look for clues that might give you more information.

You sit down in Mrs Baker's immaculate front room. There are family pictures all around the room. She has made a pot of tea and there is a plate of biscuits set down for you. She sighs in some discomfort and thanks you for coming over.

How should you begin your consultation?

This consultation should begin with an open question, such as, 'Tell me about the problem' or, 'How can I help you, Mrs Baker?' You can then clarify this with some further closed questions later. She's probably got a pretty good idea about what you need to know.

What specific questions will you need to ask?

You should find out about:
- the story of the **pain itself**, such as what (if anything) set it off, its duration, severity
- how this pain is affecting her life, such as her **mobility** and her **ability to do things**
- whether she has taken anything for the pain.

Mrs Baker tells you that it started when she reached up to get something from the kitchen cupboard. The pain is worse when she uses her arm a lot and if she has to walk a long distance with her Zimmer. She tells you she finds it difficult stretching up to get dressed. She hasn't tried anything yet for the pain.

What is your differential diagnosis? Suggest three possibilities.

- Mechanical strain (including muscle strain).
- Frozen shoulder.
- Shoulder OA.
- Tendonitis.

Examination

You ask to examine Mrs Brown's shoulder, and she takes off her jumper. It is at this point that you notice some significant areas of bruising all down her right arm up to the shoulder joint. Through her light slip you can also detect some large areas of bruising across her back. She sees you noticing this and she begins to cry.

What are your thoughts now?

Mrs Baker hasn't mentioned any history of falling. Her bruising may be concerning and needs to be explored further.

How do you proceed?

You should continue gently and sympathetically. Mrs Baker will hopefully tell you more if she feels she can trust you and if you listen to what she has to say. Give her time and space to talk.

Mrs Baker holds back the tears for a second and apologises. You ask her gently about the bruising and she tells you that this happened a couple of weeks ago when she was getting out of the bath. Her daughter was helping her, but they started arguing with each other. June got frustrated and pushed Mrs Baker back. Mrs Baker fell over, knocking her arm and back against the bath and the sink.

Mrs Baker goes on to say that June is not very happy at the moment. She has a lot of stress at work and she worries that this and being her carer is taking its toll. She has never pushed her over before, but she has often shouted 'mean things' to her mum. This upsets Mrs Baker a lot and she starts crying again. She also says that when June is really fed up with her she doesn't give her dinner in the evening.

What are you thoughts as to what is going on now?

You should be concerned that Mrs Baker is now being subjected to elder abuse. There is a history of an episode of **physical abuse** and a story of likely **emotional abuse** and possible **neglect**.

Types of elder abuse

Elder abuse is defined as a knowing, intentional, or negligent act to a vulnerable adult:
- physical abuse
- emotional abuse
- financial/exploitative abuse
- sexual abuse
- neglect or abandonment
- institutional abuse
- discriminatory abuse.

General Practice Cases at a Glance, First Edition. Carol Cooper and Martin L Block. © 2017 John Wiley & Sons, Ltd. Published 2017 by John Wiley & Sons, Ltd.

What other areas should you explore?

It is probably worth gently exploring each of the above areas, as well as finding out whether there have been any other episodes of physical abuse.

Mrs Baker tells you that is all. She is worried that if June finds out about her talking about this that she will get angry.

Who should you be contacting for more advice?

This would be a good case to discuss with the **Adult Safeguarding Team** in your local Social Services.

You tell Mrs Baker that you would like to involve this team and she agrees. You pass on Mrs Baker's details to them and they agree to visit and assess later that afternoon. The Adult Safeguarding Team will assess the level of risk to Mrs Baker and work with her to ensure that she is safe. It is likely that this discussion will extend to other family members, and as her GP you may be involved in the process (e.g. writing reports, attending a case conference). Maintaining your trusting relationship with Mrs Baker will be a foundation of this.

Finally, do not forget to talk about pain relief. Mrs Baker would benefit from trying some simple analgesia such as paracetamol in the first instance.

Resources

Age UK: Advice on elder abuse.
   http://www.ageuk.org.uk/health-wellbeing/relationships-and-family/protecting-yourself/what-is-elder-abuse/

CASE 9

I can't believe how much weight I've put on

Yvonne Green, age 39 years
Administrator
PMH: TOP; depression age 24
Medication: none

Ms Green is concerned because her weight has gone up nearly 10 kg in about a year. She says she is 5'6" (1.68 m) tall and now weighs 84 kg. She works in admin at a car hire company. Her previous medical history includes a termination at 18 and an episode of depression at 24. She has no children.

She has tried 'everything' including fat-binding tablets and a special herbal tea. Now she says, 'You've got me to help me, doctor.'

What is overweight or obese?

World Health Organization (WHO) states that for adults, the healthy range for BMI is between 18.5 and 24.9.
- **Overweight:** BMI greater than or equal to 25 is overweight.
- **Obesity:** BMI greater than or equal to 30 is obesity.
With the rise in extreme obesity, there are now additional categories.
- **Super-obesity:** BMI greater than or equal to 50.
- **Super-super-obesity:** BMI greater than or equal to 60.
N.B. BMI can be misleadingly high in very muscular people.

What are your initial thoughts?

You suspect she is eating too much and exercising too little, but 10 kg is a lot in a relatively short period of time and it's important to rule out medical causes for her weight gain, especially common treatable conditions like polycystic ovary syndrome (PCOS) and hypothyroidism.

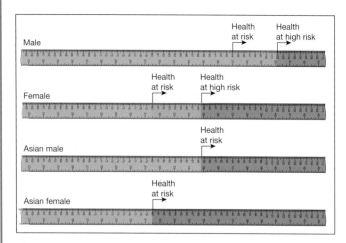

Figure 9.1 Waist size and health: what is known.

Some causes of overweight/weight gain

Common
- Eating too much/exercising too little.
- Depression.
- Eating disorder.
- Type 2 diabetes.
- Hypothyroidism.
- Pregnancy.
- PCOS.
- Menopause.
- Drugs, including steroids, antipsychotics, antidepressants (especially tricyclics), antihypertensives (especially betablockers), contraceptive pill. Statins may also be linked with weight gain as those taking them can become less fat-conscious and take in more calories.

Less common
- Fluid retention from nephrotic syndrome or liver disease.
- Cushing's disease.
- Acromegaly.
- Frontal lobe brain tumour (causing hyperphagia).
- Benign intracranial hypertension.
- Post-encephalitis weight gain.

What useful questions could you ask? Write down at least five.

- 'How are **things generally**?' This is a good opener for talking about depression and other things, though in the light of her past history you could consider being more direct.
- 'What **exercise** do you do?' Her work is sedentary so try to establish how active she is outside work.
- 'Has **anything changed** lately?' This could be anything, from getting free meals at work to recent marriage, a known cause of weight gain in both partners.
- 'When was your last **period**?' This is a key question for PCOS and the menopause. Pregnancy is less likely here as weight gain has occurred over 12 months.
- Establish whether there's a **family history** of weight problems, diabetes and thyroid disease. If she doesn't know what the thyroid is, it's likely that no close relative has thyroid trouble.
- 'Have you any **other symptoms**?' You could prompt her by mentioning skin changes (Cushing's, PCOS), body hair (PCOS), facial appearance (thyroid disease, Cushing's). The trouble with mentioning headaches (intracranial hypertension) is that so many people have them.

She has no other symptoms. Her periods have 'always' been irregular. She can't recall her LMP but it was in the last two months. She is not on the contraceptive pill or any other drugs. Her life is not very active, and the only recent change is that she moved into a flat with a lift.

Nobody in her family is especially large, and there's no diabetes. One aunt had thyroid trouble. She is not sure about her mother who died young.

Do you examine her? If so, what do you look for?

- Take note of her general **demeanour and affect** (depression) and her physical appearance (Cushing's, hypothyroidism, hirsutism).
- Her **weight** and **waist circumference** will be useful to monitor her progress.
- Check her **BP**.
- You might want to examine her neck (autoimmune thyroiditis).
- Consider **urine dipstick** for glucose and protein, and perhaps a pregnancy test.

You could do a lot more, including checking for striae and other hallmarks of Cushing's. But examining every single overweight patient can take up a lot of consulting time without much return.

Her affect and her face appear normal, and her BP is 146/93. She weighs 85 kg today, and her waist is 92 cm. You calculate her BMI to be 30.1. Urine dipstick is normal.

Hypothyroidism

- Affects 2% of women, 0.1% of men.
- Diagnosis: high TSH and low free T4, with or without clinical signs/symptoms.
- In 'subclinical hypothyroidism' (about 8% of women, 3% men) there are usually no symptoms, and TSH is high with a normal T4, confirmed on repeat testing after at least three months.
- Features of hypothyroidism can take years to appear, and diagnosis is often made late.
- More from CKS/NICE (see Resources).

What are your thoughts now? Write down three possibilities.

- PCOS.
- Type 2 diabetes.
- Hypothyroidism.
- An early menopause is also possible. This often runs in families.

Which investigations do you consider?

- Fasting **lipid** profile.
- **Liver** function tests.
- **Thyroid** function tests.
- Fasting glucose and **haemoglobin A1c** (HbA1c).
- **LH**, **FSH** and **testosterone** levels.

What else do you need to do for this patient?

- Bring her back to have her blood pressure checked as well as to discuss her blood test results.
- Warn her that so-called slimming remedies are a waste of money, and some can be harmful.

When she returns the following week, her blood pressure is 146/82 and her results are available (Table 9.1).

What is the diagnosis?

She has hypothyroidism.

What do you do now?

Prescribe levothyroxine. You can start on 50 or even 100 µg a day as she is young and otherwise well, but, in elderly patients and those with ischaemic heart disease, begin with a small dose, e.g. 12.5–25 µg daily.

CS9 Table 1 Blood test results for Ms Green.

	Value	Reference range
Total cholesterol	5.0 mmol/L	5.0 mmol/L or less
LDL cholesterol	2.9 mmol/L	3.0 mmol/L or less
HDL	2.0 mmol/L	> 1 mmol/L
Fasting triglycerides	0.8 mmol/L	< 1.7 mmol/L
ALT	10 U/L	5–45 U/L
GGT	34 U/L	<65 U/L
Total bilirubin	1.3 µmol/L	1–10 µmol/L
TSH	13 mU/L	0.4–4.5 mU/L
Free thyroxine (FT4)	1.8 pmol/L	3.5–7.8 pmol/L
Total tri-iodothyronine (T3)	1.4 nmol/L	1.2–2.6 nmol/L
Fasting glucose	4.6 mmol/L	<6.1 mmol/L Impaired glucose tolerance 6.1–6.9 mmol/L; diabetes ≥7.0 mmol/L
Hba1c	31 mmol/mol	Non-diabetes 20–41 mmol/mol
LH	9 IU/L	0.5–14.5 IU/L follicular and luteal phase 16–84 IU/L ovulation 17–75 IU/L postmenopausal
FSH	10 IU/L	1–11 IU/L follicular and luteal phase 6–26 IU/L ovulation 30–118 IU/L postmenopausal
Testosterone	0.9 nmol/L	<1.8 nmol/L for adult female

Clinical benefits begin within five days and level off after 4–6 weeks, so check TFTs again then. Note that TSH may take months to drop to normal. Changes to the dose of levothyroxine should be made every 6–8 weeks or so if needed, until TSH is in the target range.

If she is planning on conceiving, you may need to treat her more aggressively.

Can you assure her that all the weight will come off when her thyroid is under control?

No. She should lose weight, but may not attain her target weight simply by taking thyroxine tablets. Consider exercise referral and dietary advice.

Resources

NICE guideline CG43 Obesity: guidance on the prevention, identification, assessment and management of overweight and obesity in adults in children.
http://www.nice.org.uk/guidance/cg43/chapter/appendix-d-existing-guidance-on-diet-physical-activity-and-preventing-obesity

CKS/NICE Hypothyroidism.
http://cks.nice.org.uk/hypothyroidism

NICE: PCOS – metformin in women not planning to conceive.
http://www.nice.org.uk/advice/esuom6

RCOG: Long-term consequences of PCOS.
https://www.rcog.org.uk/globalassets/documents/guidelines/gtg-33-pcos-2014.pdf

CASE

10 It's my back passage

Ron Johnson, age 63 years
Retired maintenance engineer
PMH: COPD; accident at work
Medication: ipratropium and salbutamol inhalers

Ron Johnson has pain in his back passage. He's not sure exactly how long he's had it but it's there when he opens his bowels, and he's also seen a bit of blood lately. His previous history includes two operations on his leg following an accident. He still smokes despite COPD.

Causes of anal pain

- Anal fissure (usually pain only on defecation, but there may be a slight after-burn).
- Thrombosed external pile (note that uncomplicated haemorrhoids are painless).
- Ano-genital warts (usually painless, but can burn).
- Herpes.
- Other STIs affecting the rectum: chlamydia, gonorrhoea, syphilis.
- Skin infections: yeasts, fungi and bacteria.
- Fistula-in-ano.
- Proctalgia fugax (thought to be due to muscle spasm, it can produce a very sharp pain that often resolves quickly – occurs in both men and women).
- Levator ani syndrome (also thought to be due to muscle spasm, and more common in women).
- Skin condition: eczema or psoriasis.
- Coccydynia.
- Rectal foreign body.
- Prostatitis.

What questions might you ask him now about his symptoms? Write down at least four.

- 'When do you get the pain?' Ask the usual questions (SOCRATES) to find out more, and establish whether there's itching.
- 'Is the blood in the toilet **pan, on the paper,** or **in the motions**?' You need to ask slowly and clearly, and maybe more than once as it's a complex question. Many patients reply 'Both', not realizing there are three possible answers.
- 'Have your **bowels changed** lately?' Constipation causes hard stools and is one common reason for painful defecation, as are loose stools. Try to establish if Mr Johnson has a ► change in bowel habit which may need attention in its own right. It's also useful to know if he habitually strains when sitting on the toilet.
- 'What have you tried already?' This is a good question for most symptoms as patients may have already tried over-the-counter remedies. Occasionally an open question like this one will reveal

bizarre and harmful toilet habits, such as the use of implements to help evacuation, which can of course cause pain and bleeding. Patients are reluctant to volunteer this type of information and need to feel at ease first so it's best to ask this question last.

Mr Johnson's pain doesn't radiate anywhere, and nothing seems to relieve it. He is not too sure where the blood is; he thinks in the pan. He doesn't strain more than 'the normal amount'. He then embarks on a long story about redecorating the bathroom recently, which doesn't seem very relevant. You finally establish that his bowels haven't really changed. If they had, you'd need to ask about:

- **recent travel** (gastroenteritis)
- ► **weight loss** (carcinoma)
- **family history** of any bowel problems include cancer and polyps.

He did go to the pharmacist and bought some cream which cost more than he'd expected and didn't help. His wife told him to stop messing with expensive stuff and to come to the doctor and get a prescription. She thinks he's entitled to something back from the NHS. By now you are running very late.

Do you examine him?

Yes. Anal pain is a symptom of many different conditions and you can't tell from the history which one your patient has. He also has bleeding, and this should be taken seriously, except perhaps in a younger patient who only has blood on the paper.

Causes of rectal bleeding

- Haemorrhoids.
- Anal fissure.
- Gastroenteritis.
- Colorectal cancer.
- Inflammatory bowel disease (e.g. Crohn's or ulcerative colitis).
- Anal cancer.
- Sexually transmitted diseases.
- Anorectal trauma.Colonic polyps.
- Diverticular disease (any bleeding is usually brisk).
- Angiodysplasia of the colon.
- Ischaemic colitis.

The higher the source, the more likely the blood is to be mixed with the motion and may be dark. However a brisk upper GI bleed can cause bright red blood PR. Sources lower down usually produce bright red blood on the paper, or sometimes in the pan. Haemorrhoids typically cause bleeding in the pan.

On examination you see a sentinel pile and his anus is in spasm so you abandon digital rectal examination.

What do you prescribe?

There's a range of prescribable **local anaesthetic preparations** in the BNF, such as Proctosedyl. For anal fissure you can also prescribe Rectogesic which contains glyceryl trinitrate. You can also advise him to eat bran, or try a bulking agent like ispaghula husk (Fybogel) to **soften the stool**.

Ten days later he is back. The pain is worse, and sometimes it hurts to sit. He wants something stronger on prescription and gives you the same story about his entitlement to free prescriptions. And you are running late again.

What do you do now?

Examine him again. His main symptom is pain, which is not settling, and is no longer limited to defecation.

>
> **Tip**
> Surgeons often say that if you don't put your finger in it, you put your foot in it. The adage still holds true in primary care, and shortage of time should never be an excuse for substandard care.

This time you do a PR and are surprised to find a craggy ulcer on one side of the anal canal, within easy reach of your examining finger.

Is there anything else you could do?

• You could palpate his **liver** and feel for **inguinal lymph nodes**, though inguinal node enlargement is often misleading (it can occur through walking barefoot).
• You could also find out more about his **sexual practices**, though this is not of great practical use as your findings need treatment in their own right. If you do, ask if he has ever had sex with another man, rather than asking if he is gay.

Now what do you do?

Refer him to the colorectal service under the two-week rule. While anal cancer is rare, it is a possibility that needs to be ruled out. You can tell him that he has an ulcer in his back passage, which is the likely cause of his pain. You're not sure how serious it is, but it's not something that can be dealt with in general practice, so you're sending him to a specialist within two weeks to make sure.

> **Rectal bleeding: two-week wait referral criteria for suspected cancer**
>
> • ▶ Age ≥50 years with unexplained rectal bleeding.
> • ▶ Age <50 years with rectal bleeding and any of the following: abdominal pain; change in bowel habit; weight loss; iron-deficiency anaemia.
> • ▶ Rectal bleeding and a palpable rectal mass.
> (adapted from NICE guidelines NG12)

Post-script: Mr Johnson turns out to have anal carcinoma. In her letter, the surgeon tells you she hopes to excise it via a sphincter-sparing procedure.

Carcinoma of the anus

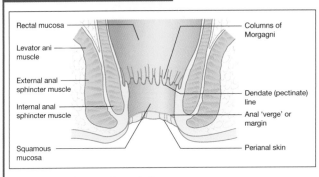

Figure 10.1 Section through the anus.

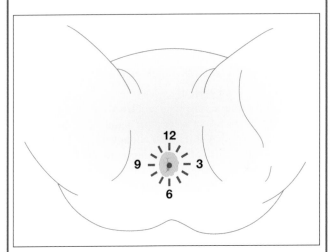

Figure 10.2 Describing the position of anal lesions.

In the UK only 1000 people a year are diagnosed with it. The most common type is squamous cell carcinoma (80%). Other types include basal cell carcinoma and adenocarcinoma.

Symptoms
• Sometimes none.
• ▶ PR bleeding.
• Pain or itching.
• Mucous discharge.
• ▶ Incontinence from sphincter involvement.
• Perianal ulcers or lumps.

Risk factors
• Women slightly more than men.
• HPV infection.
• Receptive anal sex.
• HIV and other immune deficiencies.
• Smoking.

Resources

CKS/NICE guidance: Suspected cancer: recognition and referral. http://www.nice.org.uk/guidance/conditions-and-diseases/cancer
You may also like to try Case 41: 'I'm having terrible diarrhoea'.

CASE
11 I am pregnant again

Mrs Hoda Ibrahim, age 29 years
Housewife
PMH: none
Medication: none

Mrs Hoda Ibrahim is from Somalia and her pregnancy test is positive. Her three other children were born abroad. Her last pregnancy and birth were 'very difficult' and baby was small. There is no other history available.

What do you ask? List three or four vital questions.

• 'When was your last **period**?'
• 'Did anyone in your **family** have problems in pregnancy?' You're after a history of pre-eclampsia or other significant problems.
• 'Do you take **any medicines**?' Ask about vitamins/herbs too.
• '**Were you cut**?' This is the best direct question about female genital mutilation (FGM) but it helps to begin with a statement: 'We know cutting happens to girls and women in many countries.'

FGM

Widespread in Africa and the Middle East, FGM is a cultural practice, not religious. In Somalia almost all girls have FGM. It can be done at any age and have lifelong repercussions.
Obstetric complications
• fear of pregnancy and labour
• difficult vaginal examinations in labour
• difficulty with scalp electrodes and fetal blood sampling
• C-section
• episiotomy or tear
• fistula
• postpartum haemorrhage.

Hoda's LMP was 23 July with a regular cycle, making her due on April 15, and she is now 10 weeks pregnant. She was cut when she was 11. She does not want you to examine her there but lets you check her abdomen, heart and lungs, which are all normal. BP is 95/60. She thinks it was higher in her last pregnancy, and her sister also had high blood pressure.

Do you need to examine her perineum or do a vaginal examination?

No, as this will be done at the hospital. Give advice about safe eating in pregnancy and prescribe **folic acid** 400 µg daily and **vitamin D** as 400 U/10 µg colecalciferol daily.

What other important areas should you cover in this consultation?

• You might already have clues from her body language, but find out how she feels. Being married does not mean this pregnancy is

welcome. Avoid leading questions. Something like 'Are you happy about being pregnant?' should work.
• What does her **family** think of a new baby? Her partner may be less pleased. Domestic violence is more common in pregnancy.
• Are family near? Any **support** she gets from family can mean less of a burden on social care.

Apart from her LMP and BMI, what two points should you mention in your referral to antenatal?

• **FGM.** You may not know what type she had, but flag it up so she gets a full assessment before labour (see Figure 11.1).
• Possible **pre-eclampsia** in her last pregnancy, and her sister's. You next see Hoda at 33 weeks with pain and tingling in her fingers. It is between antenatal visits and she has not brought her patient-held notes but she says the pregnancy is 'good'. The hospital has suggested a vaginal delivery with an epidural.

You suspect carpal tunnel syndrome and tell her it will get better. You check her BP and urine, which are due next week. BP is 136/90 and she has 1+ of protein in her urine.

Which of these do you do now?

(a) Nothing.
(b) Give her medication for her BP.
(c) Refer her to hospital.
(c) is correct. Her blood pressure is significantly raised (diastolic 90 or more) and she has proteinuria. She may have pre-eclampsia, so you should refer her to the antenatal clinic or day assessment unit today.

Key point

Every doctor who deals with pregnant women must know how to deal with this kind of scenario. There are still avoidable maternal deaths from pre-eclampsia in the UK, and around 1000 babies die from the condition.

Hoda reluctantly goes to hospital where her BP settles. She returns next week because her baby seems to be moving less. BP is 133/86 and she still has 1+ proteinuria.

What do you do now?

(a) Tell her to come back tomorrow or the day after.
(b) Tell her it is normal for babies to move less as the womb has less space towards the end of pregnancy.
(c) Refer to hospital again.
Hoda's BP is lower today, but she has proteinuria and symptoms so it's (c). Refer her back to hospital today as per the guidelines. Reduced fetal movement is a symptom of fetal compromise.

Tip

Always listen to a pregnant woman who tells you her baby is moving less. Remember too that pre-eclampsia does not always mean raised BP. There can be proteinuria alone.

General Practice Cases at a Glance, First Edition. Carol Cooper and Martin L Block. © 2017 John Wiley & Sons, Ltd. Published 2017 by John Wiley & Sons, Ltd.

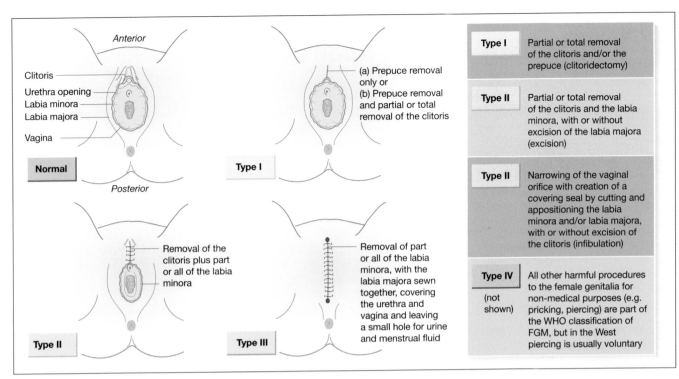

Figure 11.1 Types of FGM (from WHO classification).

Table 11.1 Dealing with new hypertension and/or proteinuria after 20 weeks (from PRECOG, the pre-eclampsia community guideline).

Description	Definition	Action by midwife/GP	Description	Definition	Action by midwife/GP
New hypertension without proteinuria after 20 weeks	Diastolic BP ≥ 90 and < 100 mmHg	Refer for hospital assessment within 48 hours	New hypertension without hypertension after 20 weeks	1+ on dipstick	Repeat pre-eclampsia assessment in community within 1 week
	Diastolic BP ≥ 90 and < 100 mmHg with significant symptoms*	Refer for same day hospital assessment		2+ or more on dipstick	Refer for hospital assessment within 48 hours
	Systolic BP ≥ 160 mmHg	Refer for same day hospital assessment		≥1+ on dipstick with significant symptoms*	Refer for same day hospital assessment
	Diastolic BP ≥ 100 mmHg	Refer for same day hospital assessment	Maternal symptoms or fetal signs and symptoms without new hypertension or proteinuria	Headache and/or visual disturbances with diastolic blood pressure less than 90 mmHg and a trace or no protein	Follow local protocols for investigation. Consider reducing interval before next assessment
New hypertension and proteinuria after 20 weeks	Diastolic BP ≥ 90 mmHg and new proteinuria ≥1+ on dipstick	Refer for same day hospital assessment		Epigastric pain with diastolic blood pressure less than 90 mmHg and a trace or no protein	Refer for same day hospital assessment
	Diastolic BP ≥ 110 mmHg and new proteinuria ≥1+ on dipstick	Arrange immediate admission		Reduced movements or small for gestational age infant with diastolic blood pressure less than 90 mmHg and a trace or no protein	Follow local protocols for investigation of fetal compromise. Consider reducing interval before next full pre-eclampsia assessment
	Systolic BP ≥ 170 mmHg and new proteinuria ≥1+ on dipstick	Arrange immediate admission			
	Diastolic BP ≥ 90 mmHg and new proteinuria ≥1+ on dipstick and significant symptoms*	Arrange immediate admission			

*Epigastric pain, vomiting, headache, visual disturbances, reduced fetal movements, small for gestational age infant

Two months later you see Hoda with a healthy baby girl.

What more can you do for her and her family?

- Discuss **contraception**.
- Check her **BP again at six weeks**.
- Talk about the dangers of subjecting her children to cutting. FGM is also illegal under the FGM Act 2003.
- Encourage her to bring her baby for routine **check-ups** and **immunizations**.

Resources
CKS/NICE Hypertension in pregnancy.
  http://cks.nice.org.uk/hypertension-in-pregnancy
CKS/NICE Antenatal care – uncomplicated pregnancy.
  http://cks.nice.org.uk/antenatal-care-uncomplicated-pregnancy
FGM in pregnancy.
  https://www.rcog.org.uk/globalassets/documents/guidelines/greentop53femalegenitalmutilation.pdf
The FGM Act 2003.
  http://www.legislation.gov.uk/ukpga/2003/31/contents

CASE

12 My baby has an upset tummy

Shanti Patel, age 6 months
PMH: nil
Medication: nil

Six-month-old Shanti is brought to the surgery because she has been vomiting since yesterday afternoon. For three days now she has had diarrhoea. On questioning, her mother tells you that the baby has loose runny poo, up to six or seven times a day, and it leaks out of the nappy. She seems a bit grumpy compared to usual, and is taking less milk. She is bottle-fed and all her immunizations are up to date. There is one older brother.

What are your priorities in this consultation? Write down at least three objectives.

• Establish whether this is **gastroenteritis**, as it appears to be, or something else. Diarrhoea and vomiting can occur in young children with other conditions, such as intussusception and septicaemia (sepsis).
• Assess whether Shanti is **dehydrated**.
• Manage the **symptoms**.
• If it's gastroenteritis, prevent its **spread**. Note that food-poisoning and dystentery (diarrhoea with blood and mucus) are **notifiable**. You ask more about the symptoms, and learn that there is no blood in the poo and no bile in the vomit. The mother can't tell if Shanti's nappies are drier than usual.

Conditions that can mimic gastroenteritis

• Children can have diarrhoea or vomiting when they have **other infections**, such as UTI, otitis media, chest infection, meningitis, septicaemia (sepsis).
• Other **abdominal conditions** can cause similar symptoms: pyloric stenosis, intussusception, coeliac disease, gastro-oesophageal reflux.
• Older children may have constipation with **overflow**.
• **Diabetic keto-acidosis** can cause D&V, and can be the first presentation of diabetes in a child.

What else should you ask? Write down three or four questions.

• Is Shanti having **solids**, and if so what? The recommended weaning age on to solid food in the UK is six months, but many parents start much earlier.
• Has there been **contact** with someone with similar symptoms?
• Has there been foreign **travel**? This is usually linked with infectious gastroenteritis, including parasitic infestations, but Ebola fever can also begin with diarrhoea.
• Has the baby had any **medication** and has the mother tried any remedies yet? Some parents give oral rehydration solution, others try fizzy drinks or alternative treatments. This line of questioning can also uncover recent antibiotics prescribed by another doctor (or given by a relative), which the parent may not otherwise reveal.

Mrs Patel tells you that the older brother fleetingly had tummy ache last night but is well. There have been no other contacts, and no travel. Shanti has not had any medicine but Mrs Patel has diluted Shanti's formula feeds since yesterday. She is not having solid food.

You examine Shanti.

Write down at least three red flag signs which might suggest this is not gastroenteritis.

➤ High fever (greater or equal to 39 °C in children over 3 months, greater or equal to 38 °C in babies under 3 months).
➤ Bulging fontanelle.
➤ Abdominal distension.
➤ Rash, especially if non-blanching, would also suggest this is not gastroenteritis.

And what are the red flag signs of dehydration? Write down at least six.

➤ Altered responsiveness (irritability or lethargy).
➤ Increased capillary refill time (greater than 3 seconds).
➤ Sunken eyes.
➤ Sunken fontanelle.
➤ Tachycardia (HR >160/min if under 12 months; >150/min if 12–24 months old; >140/min if 2–5 years old).
➤ Tachypnoea (RR >60/min if under 6 months; >50/min if 6–12 months; > 40/min for children over 12 months).
➤ Cold extremities.
➤ Pale or mottled skin.

Shanti's temperature is 37.6 °C. She is a bit grumpy but has no other signs of dehydration. Her HR is 140 and her abdomen is normal. She has a nappy rash. Overall she does not appear very ill to you, and she seems about the right size and developmental stage for her age. You suspect it is gastroenteritis.

Do you need a stool specimen?

No. In general, you only need to send a stool sample to the lab if:
• there's been recent travel
• diarrhoea persists for more than six days
• you're not sure of the diagnosis
• it's an outbreak of gastroenteritis
• the child is immunocompromised.

🔑 Key point

The clinical priority is the same here, regardless of the cause of gastroenteritis: prevent or treat dehydration.

Shanti is not dehydrated now, but some children are at **increased risk of dehydration**:
• babies under 12 months old, especially those under six months
• passing more than five loose stools in 24 hours
• vomiting more than twice in 24 hours
• unable to keep down rehydration fluids
• babies who were of low birthweight or malnourished
• weaned off the breast during their illness.

General Practice Cases at a Glance, First Edition. Carol Cooper and Martin L Block. © 2017 John Wiley & Sons, Ltd. Published 2017 by John Wiley & Sons, Ltd.

Childhood gastroenteritis

Gastroenteritis is very common. Every year, about 10% of children under five present to a doctor with it, and many more episodes are treated without involving medical help.

The cause can be **viral**, **bacterial** or **parasitic**.

Common organisms in UK
- rotavirus (was the most common cause but recent introduction of oral vaccine may change this)
- *Campylobacter*
- *Salmonella*
- *Shigella*
- norovirus
- *E. coli*.

Bloody diarrhoea is most likely with *Campylobacter* and *E. coli*.

Poor hygiene increases the risk.

Breast-feeding confers some protection as it eliminates the risk of transmission via feeding equipment, and also transmits antibodies from the mother (breast milk also contains lymphocytes).

Most cases improve without the organism being identified. Diarrhoea usually resolves within 5–7 days, and in most cases stops by 14 days. Vomiting usually resolves within 1–2 days, and in most cases stops by three days.

Complications of gastroenteritis
- dehydration
- haemolytic–uraemic syndrome
- loss of lactase from the gut, causing temporary lactose intolerance.

Stool colour is not always important. If a child is well, green stools don't matter. Infant motions come in an array of colours, most of them normal. The exceptions to note are:
- red (blood)
- black (altered blood)
- chalky white (bile duct obstruction).

What advice do now you give Mrs Patel? Write down four recommendations.

- Continue with milk feeds.
- Add oral rehydration solution (not fruit juice or soft drinks). Shanti is not clinically dehydrated now, but she is at risk of becoming so.
- She should wash her hands with soap and water after changing nappies, and keep the baby's things, including towels and toys, separate from the rest of the family.
- Bring her baby back the next day for review, or earlier if there are symptoms/signs of dehydration such as drowsiness, clammy or mottled skin, or decreased urine; or if the baby continues to vomit (this suggests she is not absorbing anything by mouth). It is worth spending some time explaining to Mrs Patel what to look out for.

Managing gastroenteritis in children

Management involves the replacement of lost fluids. It's rare to have to treat the underlying cause.

Don't use antidiarrhoeal agents.

For gastroenteritis without dehydration
- continue breast or bottle feeds
- encourage clear fluids, but not fruit juice or fizzy drinks
- use oral rehydration solution for those at higher risk of dehydration.

Treating dehydration
- use oral rehydration solution unless IV treatment is needed
- give often and in small amounts – a child needs 50 ml/kg over 4 hours to replace fluid
- reassess clinically to monitor the response.

Antibiotics are needed for:
- confirmed septicaemia (sepsis)
- *Salmonella* infection in the very young or the immunocompromised
- for *C. difficile*, giardiasis, bacillary or amoebic dysentery, cholera – consult a specialist first.

Key point

If you are considering food poisoning, remember this is a notifiable disease. A Notifiable Diseases form should be completed and forwarded on to Public Health who will in turn follow up.

List of notifiable diseases

Diseases notifiable to local authority proper officers under the Health Protection (Notification) Regulations 2010.
- Acute encephalitis.
- Acute infectious hepatitis.
- Acute meningitis.
- Acute poliomyelitis.
- Anthrax.
- Botulism.
- Brucellosis.
- Cholera.
- Diphtheria.
- Enteric fever (typhoid or paratyphoid fever).
- Food poisoning.
- Haemolytic–uraemic syndrome (HUS).
- Infectious bloody diarrhoea.
- Invasive group A streptococcal disease.
- Legionnaires' disease.
- Leprosy.
- Malaria.
- Measles.
- Meningococcal septicaemia.
- Mumps.
- Plague.
- Rabies.
- Rubella.
- Severe acute respiratory syndrome (SARS).
- Scarlet fever.
- Smallpox.
- Tetanus.
- Tuberculosis.
- Typhus.
- Viral haemorrhagic fever (VHF).
- Whooping cough.
- Yellow fever.

It's a statutory duty to notify these diseases. This list is not exhaustive: you must report other diseases that may present significant risk to human health under the category 'other significant disease'.

Resources

CKS/NICE Gastro-enteritis.
  http://cks.nice.org.uk/gastroenteritis
Notifiable diseases and causative organisms: how to report.
  https://www.gov.uk/notifiable-diseases-and-causative-organisms-how-to-report
You might also like to try Case 41: 'I'm having terrible diarrhoea'.

Comfort Akinsola, age 44 years
Full-time mum
PMH: fibroids
Medication: nil

Mrs Akinsola, her husband and her three children are all registered at the practice. Today Mrs Akinsola has booked in to see you in an emergency appointment. You see her sitting in the waiting room looking stony faced and call her into your consulting room.

When you ask what you can do for her today, she says, 'My ear really hurts. I am in terrible pain.' You ask her to tell you a little more about the pain, and she goes on to say, 'It really is a terrible pain. It started yesterday and got worse in the night. What can I do to make things better, doctor?'

What questions would you like to ask next? Write down four.

- 'Tell me more about the **pain**?'
- 'Do you have any **other symptoms**, such as cough or cold?'
- 'Any **fever**?' This would suggest infection.
- 'How's your **hearing**?' Hearing can be impaired in otitis media and in cases of otitis externa that lead to a build-up of debris or discharge in the canal.
- 'Any **discharge** from the ear?' This could be from a perforated drum due to otitis media or due to severe otitis externa.
- 'Do you have any **idea** what could be causing the pain?'

She tells you that the pain is a sharp, throbbing pain in her right ear. Her pinna is tender to touch. She has not had any other symptoms and no fever. She thinks her hearing is a little bit reduced on her right side. There has been no discharge. She goes swimming a lot with her children, and remembers Joshua (her youngest) splashing a lot of water in her ear earlier in the week. She wonders if this might have introduced the infection. She tried cleaning out any infection with some cotton buds, but this has not made things any better.

What is the most likely diagnosis?

So far, everything points to otitis externa (see Table 13.1 for more information).

What do you do next in the consultation?

It's time to examine the patient. You should check her temperature and examine her ear using an otoscope, ideally in the good ear. You should also assess for the presence of an upper respiratory tract infection by checking her throat, nose, cervical nodes and chest.

You examine Mrs Akinsola. Her right tragus is tender and the examination of her right ear is uncomfortable. Mrs Akinsola winces several times as you examine her. You find that her right ear canal is red and swollen and there are small amounts of debris sitting in the canal. Her drum is unaffected. Her left ear is normal. Her chest is clear, there are no swollen cervical nodes, her throat is normal and her temperature is 36.1 °C.

What is the diagnosis?

Mrs Akinsola has otitis externa (Table 13.1).

Table 13.1 Acute ear pain: otitis externa vs. infective otitis media.

Condition	Clinical findings, causes
Otitis externa: infection of ear canal	Tender tragus/pinna Canal swollen, red, tender or exudative on examination Typically caused by external organisms multiplying in ear canal, e.g. introduced in water (swimming, syringing) or introduction on dirty fingers, cotton buds
Infective otitis media: infection of middle ear	Painful inside ear Discharge only if drum perforates Red ear drum on examination Typically follows viral upper respiratory tract infection

What is the likely cause?

It is possible that the water splashed into her ear by Joshua could have brought this on. Using cotton buds internally could have made things worse and should always be actively discouraged. Sometimes the cause is not clear.

How would you explain the diagnosis?

You should use simple terms. Give Mrs Akinsola an explanation such as, 'You have an infection in the ear canal. This is the tube that links the ear on the outside with the internal ear. It's possible that the water splashed into the ear has caused the infection, and it may have been aggravated by using cotton buds.'

What should your management plan and advice be? Suggest three things.

- Topical antibiotic drops, such as Sofradex (dexamethasone sodium metasulphobenzoate /framycetin sulphate/gramicidin).
- Keep ear dry as much as possible.
- Stop using cotton buds.

Causes of otitis externa

Infections
- Bacterial (90%).
- Fungal (10%) (usually follows prolonged antibiotic treatment).
- Herpes zoster (Ramsay Hunt syndrome).

Skin conditions
- Eczema.
- Psoriasis.
- Seborrhoeic dermatitis.
- Acne.

Irritants
- Cotton buds.
- Hearing aids or earplugs.
- Foreign body.
- Polluted water (from swimming).
- Hair sprays and dyes.

What would you do in the event of treatment failure? Suggest two things.

- Swab the ear canal and send off for **culture** and **sensitivities**. Although most cases are bacterial, some are fungal.
- Refer for **micro-suction**. This will help clear the debris and hasten recovery.

General Practice Cases at a Glance, First Edition. Carol Cooper and Martin L Block. © 2017 John Wiley & Sons, Ltd. Published 2017 by John Wiley & Sons, Ltd.

CASE

14 I'm worried about my drinking

Mary McKay, age 35 years
Unemployed
PMH: acid dyspepsia
Medication: omeprazole 10 mg daily

Ms McKay has just registered at your surgery. You are seeing her for the first time today. You call her in from your waiting room and she sits down slowly with an air of sadness. You ask her what you can do for her today and she says, 'I'm worried about my drinking, doctor.'

What should you do now?

Ms McKay needs space to talk. If you interrupt during the initial 'golden minute' you may miss some important information.

You nod sympathetically and Ms McKay goes on to tell her story. 'I've always been a drinker. Right from when I was a teenager. Always enjoyed a drink. It used to be I would mostly drink at the weekends when I was out with the girls. Having a laugh. I guess things changed when I lost my job a couple of years ago. The drinking kept me sane in a way. Then I started drinking every day and it wasn't about having fun. It stopped being fun a long time ago. I drink every day now from midday through till about 11 at night. I get the cheap bottles of wine from the supermarket and get through a couple a day. It's all I can afford. I know I should stop but I'm scared to. I don't know what will happen if I do. But I know I need to. I can't continue like this.'

What else would you like ask about? Think of three things.

- **Why now**? What has made her want to stop?
- Has she tried stopping before?
- What happens if she does stop drinking? **Any physical symptoms**?
- What **support** does she have?
- Is she **depressed**?
- Does she have any thoughts of **self-harm**?

Ms McKay describes how she has a real sense that enough is enough. She thinks she realized this recently when she started shaking when she hadn't drunk till late in the day as she had a meeting at the job centre. She went home shaking and crying and cracked open a bottle of wine. This made the shakes go away. She tried stopping about a year ago, and got through a couple of weeks before she started drinking again (following an argument with her ex-partner). She is quite close to her mum, who knows about her drink problem. She had a drink problem too and she gave up about 10 years ago. She hasn't touched a drop since and advised her daughter to see her GP to get some help. She says she does get tearful, and describes how the drinking 'magnifies her emotions'. She feels that she is stuck in life and knows that if she carries on drinking like this her life will never change. She does not have thoughts of self-harm.

Where is she in the cycle of change (Figure 14.1)?

Ms McKay is here to see you because she wants help. She has therefore moved from **contemplation** to **preparation**.

Should Ms McKay stop drinking outright?

The history of withdrawal symptoms would suggest that she would benefit from a detox rather than stopping outright. She could be at risk of seizures were she to stop abruptly.

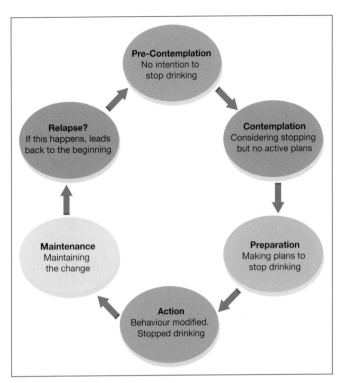

Figure 14.1 Cycle of change. Adapted from Prochaska J and DiClemente C. J Consulting & Clinical Psychology 1983; 5: 390–339.

Tip

The cycle of change is often used when thinking about patients with an addiction. It can be helpful as a guide on how to motivate people appropriately at different places in the cycle. The approach you might use for someone in the preparation phase would be very different for someone in the contemplative phase, where you might be encouraging reflection on the potential improvements a change may bring.

What should be offered to Ms McKay?

- Ms McKay should be offered an **alcohol detox**. You should have access to an alcohol worker (most likely through your local drug and alcohol team) who can talk her through the options of a community or an inpatient detox. This is achieved through a combination of psychological treatment, social support and medical treatment (e.g. short course of benzodiazepines).
- Following this she would benefit from **relapse prevention**. This can take the form of psychological therapy or larger support groups (such as Alcoholics Anonymous).
- You should give her **thiamine** 200 mg daily.

What other advice should you give Ms McKay to ensure safety?

- You should ensure she is not **driving**.
- She should not stop drinking abruptly.

Ms McKay is very keen to see the alcohol worker and start an alcohol detox as soon as possible. She is grateful that you took time to listen to her.

Resources

CKS/NICE Alcohol – problem drinking.
    http://cks.nice.org.uk/alcohol-problem-drinking

General Practice Cases at a Glance, First Edition. Carol Cooper and Martin L Block. © 2017 John Wiley & Sons, Ltd. Published 2017 by John Wiley & Sons, Ltd.

CASE

15 She cries all the time

Lily Gross, age 6 weeks
PMH: nil
Medication: nil

First-time mother Naomi Gross brings Lily in to see you, complaining that she hardly ever stops crying. Lily was born by caesarean section for fetal distress but she was fine just after the birth, and everything was going OK until about three weeks ago. It's hard for Naomi to say when the crying is worse, possibly after feeds and certainly in the evenings. She has tried everything: feeding her, rocking her, changing her, giving her water, giving her a dummy, swaddling her. Nothing seems to help. However you can't help noticing that Lily is not crying in the consulting room.

Lily is breast-fed. It took a while getting that established though it is OK now. Naomi's husband Peter helps with the baby in the evenings, when he can, but in the daytime it's just her and the baby.

What are your initial thoughts? Write down at least four possibilities.

- Normal crying and **unrealistic parental expectations**. Sometimes postnatal depression and/or a couple's relationship problems compound the issue.
- **Infant colic** (see box).
- **Reflux** (see box).
- **Teething** (unusual as early as six weeks, but possible).
- **Acute illness**, e.g. otitis media, strangulated hernia, intussusception, meningitis. These are all unlikely unless the crying is of recent or sudden onset, but illness needs to be excluded, so you will need to examine the baby.
- **Post-immunization** (babies are often fractious, but Lily has yet to have her first vaccine).

Reflux in babies

This refers to reflux of stomach contents up the oesophagus, which may or may not be linked with vomiting/excess posseting. Usually peaks between one and four months, and resolves soon after the first birthday as the gastro-oesophageal sphincter develops.

Around 40% of babies have some reflux, but in a few it causes troublesome symptoms:
- crying especially during feeds
- refusing feeds
- arching away from breast or bottle
- nocturnal cough
- failure to thrive.

Management
- holding the baby upright during feeds
- thickening the feed (if bottle-fed)
- alginate-containing preparation (e.g. Gaviscon Infant)
- H2 blockers (under specialist advice)
- PPI, e.g. omeprazole (under specialist advice).

You have a good idea of how bad the crying is and how it affects Naomi. What further questions would you like to ask?

- Are there **other symptoms**, such as diarrhoea or vomiting? Or problems with feeding? Rule out serious symptoms:

  ▶ frequent forceful (projectile) vomiting
  ▶ bile-stained vomiting
  ▶ haematemesis
  ▶ blood in the stool.

- Does Lily cry **with other adults** too?
- Are there any other **people who might give a hand**, e.g. grandparents, friends or neighbours?
- Find out if this is **getting the mother down**. You could open with 'It must be very difficult to cope with.'
- Try to ascertain **Naomi's situation**. Some factors can make parenting more difficult. Was she a high-flying professional before she had the baby? Was the pregnancy planned? Are there other worries – money, anything else?

Naomi says there are no other symptoms, and Lily feeds well. Lily does cry with other adults, but not as much. Her own mother visits at weekends – she lives a distance away. Naomi doesn't really know the neighbours yet as they are new to the area. 'Why does it all have to be so hard when you have a baby?' asks Naomi. The baby was planned, and it's all Naomi ever dreamed of. Husband Peter is a solicitor. She had a good job in advertising but is not sure she wants to return to work.

What key aims have you in mind as you examine Lily?

- Rule out **serious illness**. Look for:

  ▶ fever
  ▶ abdominal distension or mass

Colic

Around 30% of babies have colic but not everyone agrees on what it is. It may be a variant of normal crying, or it may be due to immaturity of the gut. Symptoms usually begin around two weeks and continue to 3–4 months, when they stop, either gradually or suddenly. Symptoms include:
- bouts of crying in the evenings (by definition, at least three hours' crying on at least three evenings a week, for three weeks or more)
- crying as if in pain
- pulling the legs up
- there may be noisy bowel sounds
- feeding is normal
- normal weight gain and no signs of illness
- perfectly well and happy between bouts of crying.

Management
- winding more
- anti-colic teats (if bottle-fed)
- carrying the baby on her front (over the parent's arm)
- in some cases, a dairy-free diet (if breast-feeding)
- non-dairy formula may help (if formula-fed) but don't advise swapping to a soya formula without specialist advice.

General Practice Cases at a Glance, First Edition. Carol Cooper and Martin L Block. © 2017 John Wiley & Sons, Ltd. Published 2017 by John Wiley & Sons, Ltd.

► lethargy or irritability
► bulging fontanelle.

- Assess her **growth**. ► Rapidly increasing head circumference.
- Assess her **development** (although she will still need a formal six-week check).
- Rule out **injury** (**accidental** or **non-accidental**).

On examination Lily is quiet. She does not smile at you but otherwise her development seems normal. Her HC and weight are between the 25th and 50th percentile and her length is nearer the 50th.

The baby's temperature is normal. Her chest is clear, TMs N. Abdo is normal and there are no hernias. She has no nappy rash and her mouth shows no patches of thrush. There are no signs of injury.

What are your thoughts now?

The examination has ruled out some serious problems, though not colic or reflux. The other main possibility is normal crying. Babies are not always 'settled' at six weeks, but they are very good at picking up clues. In the hands of a less experienced parent, a baby may well cry more. Naomi has 'tried everything', which is sometimes part of the problem. Babies need consistency.

What do you do?

While no dramatic action is needed here, what you do now can have a long-term effect on the family. The key is to help the mother without disempowering her. She may not be experienced, but she has spent more time with her baby than anyone else. One day, she will be the expert on her own child.

- Involve the **health visitor**, who is the professional best placed to educate and support parents of young babies.

- **Reassure and support** the parent. She is stressed, and her husband may be too. A 'difficult' baby, however you define it, increases the risk of postnatal depression, and of child abuse. It's good for her to know that other babies cry too, but choose your words carefully. 'You're not alone' may suggest that other people cope better with a crying baby than she does.
- Offer some **immediate suggestions** for her to go away with. She could try feeding the baby in an upright position to see if it helps. She could also contact the charity Cry-Sis which has a helpline for those with babies that cry excessively.
- Arrange to **review the baby** to see if her crying settles. You also need to check her social skills in a week or two. While you've already covered some of the ground in the six-week check, the baby has not smiled for you. The follow-up appointment will also be a chance for you to see how Naomi is doing and whether she is developing any features of depression. See Resources for the Edinburgh Postnatal Questionnaire.

Resources

BNF for Children.
CKS/NICE Depression – antenatal and postnatal.
  http://cks.nice.org.uk/depression-antenatal-and-postnatal
NICE Gastro-oesophageal reflux disease: recognition, diagnosis and management in children and young people.
  https://www.nice.org.uk/guidance/NG1
Cry-Sis (charity).
  www.cry-sis.org.uk/
Edinburgh Postnatal Questionnaire.
  http://www.fresno.ucsf.edu/pediatrics/downloads/edinburghscale.pdf

CASE
16   I need something to help me sleep

Sophie Henry, age 35 years

Freelance journalist
PMH: TOP; Lyme disease
Medication: oral contraceptive pill

Sophie Henry comes to see you, saying she's tried everything and still can't sleep, ending with, 'And now you need to do something.' She looks tired and a bit agitated, and she adds that lack of sleep is affecting her work.

She is self-employed, working as a freelance journalist for various magazines. Occasionally she works shifts in an office, but mostly she writes features from home. Last time she attended, she saw a doctor who said there might be something that she could try. The medical notes, made by a locum, are sketchy. While you get up to speed with her records, she adds, 'I know perfectly well that there are sleeping pills you can prescribe, but you doctors don't like pills any more.'

While you can appreciate Sophie's problem, you already feel under attack at this early stage in the consultation. Instead of pointing out your position along with the potential dangers of hypnotics, you wisely decide to start from the beginning and take a full history.

What are the two main aspects of your history-taking?

Your aim is to discover any underlying cause for her insomnia, and to establish how her symptoms affect her life. In doing so, try to build a rapport with Sophie. It looks like this may not have been the case when she saw the locum, and if you relate to her it will make the consultation more effective.

Tip

Insomnia affects at least 30% of people, and is a common symptom in general practice. Up to 70% of cases are secondary to something else, so always look for these.

Causes of insomnia

Psychosocial reasons
- Bereavement.
- Environmental causes (e.g. noise, heat).

Mental health problems
Depression, anxiety, psychoses.

Physical problems
- Cardiovascular, e.g. congestive heart failure.
- Respiratory, e.g. asthma, COPD.
- Loss of diurnal pattern, e.g. dementia, Parkinson's, head injury.
- Hyperthyroidism.
- Musculoskeletal, e.g. back pain, arthritis, restless legs, chronic fatigue syndrome.
- Gastrointestinal, e.g. colitis, IBS, reflux oesophagitis.

- Urinary, e.g. UTI, nephrotic syndrome.
- Diabetes and other causes of polyuria.
- Sleep apnoea and parasomnias.

Drugs
- Prednisolone, betablockers, sympathomimetics (theophylline, salmeterol).
- Recreational drugs (mainly stimulants).
- Alcohol (induces drowsiness but spoils sleep).
- Tobacco and e-cigarettes (nicotine is a stimulant).

What important questions do you ask her? Write down at least seven.

'Tell me more about your lack of sleep' may uncover all you need to know. On the other hand, you may need to ask a number of closed questions such as:
- 'Do you have trouble **falling asleep, staying asleep**, or do you **wake very early** in the morning?' These often have different causes.
- 'When did it all **start**?' There might have been a bereavement, or an important lifestyle change.
- 'Do you find that you're **dozy during the day**? Do you nod off at the wheel or when sitting in a chair? Do you happen to know if you **snore**?' These are key questions for sleep apnoea.
- 'Do you **nap** during the day?' This is usually counterproductive as it interferes with sleep later.
- 'What's your **bedtime routine** like?' Many people expect to fall asleep as soon as they hit the pillow, even when they've spent the evening with a laptop. If she lives with a partner, his lifestyle comes into it too.
- Get an idea of her **physical health**. Is there any pain, asthma, cardiovascular disease, nocturia? Find out how much exercise she takes.
- Remember to ask about her **mood** (important for depression).
- 'Do you take any **medicines** apart from the contraceptive pill? Or any other **drugs** at all?' Stimulants (ecstasy, amphetamines, cocaine) are most likely to cause insomnia, but any recreational drug use can be significant.
- 'Do you drink **alcohol**? Roughly how much?'
- 'Do you **smoke**?'
- 'How much **tea** and **coffee** do you drink, and when during the day?' Also ask about cola drinks and other soft drinks that contain **caffeine**. It is worth mentioning that a person's sensitivity to caffeine can change with age.

Sophie is surprised you ask so many questions but seems pleased you are taking an interest. She mainly has trouble falling asleep, and this began at least a year ago. Nothing happened then that she can recall.

She is a non-smoker but drinks 'three or four' glasses of wine a night. During the day she drinks a lot of coffee, and finishes the day with a cup of weak tea before bed. She lives with her boyfriend, and neither of them snores. Most evenings are spent at home. Apart from the Pill, she takes no drugs, and has not smoked cannabis for many years.

She went freelance two years ago and feels she has to get a good night's sleep as it's tough to make ends meet in journalism these days. She does feel sleepy during the day sometimes, but doesn't nap. There are no features of depression or any other illness. Her weight is normal, so sleep apnoea is unlikely.

- Keep the **bedroom** for sex and sleep.
- **Jot down her worries** before going to bed, and tell herself that it's tomorrow's agenda.

Sleep apnoea

An important and sometimes fatal condition.
Intermittent partial or complete upper airway obstruction causes falls in pO_2 and wakes the person from sleep.
Affects 5% or so of the general population.
Can affect both men and women, especially if obese.
Linked with fatalities on the road, and with hypertension and cardiovascular events.

Symptoms
- snoring, especially with gasping and breath-holding
- unrefreshing sleep
- daytime sleepiness, which may lead to falling asleep at the wheel, or at work.

Key questions
- Are you excessively sleepy during the day?
- Do you snore very loudly, gasp for air, or stop breathing at night? (This history usually comes from the partner.)
- Do you get morning headaches?
- Do you have a dry mouth when you wake up?

Health professionals must advise professional drivers and machine operators of the dangers of falling asleep at work. Those with sleepiness 'sufficient to impair driving' must inform DVLA.
The diagnosis is usually confirmed with sleep studies (polysomnography or pulse oximetry at night).

Sleep hygiene

All these points are part of so-called 'sleep hygiene'. 'Sleep hygiene' can rectify many of the factors that affect sleep. It includes:
- regular times for going to bed and waking up, no matter how bad that night's sleep was (and no sleeping in after a poor night's sleep)
- relaxing before going to bed
- making the sleep environment comfortable: not too hot, cold, noisy, or bright
- no napping during the day
- no caffeine, nicotine or alcohol within six hours of going to bed (some benefit from cutting out caffeine completely)
- exercise during the day (but not just before bed)
- no heavy meals late at night
- no checking mobiles at all hours; avoid even checking the clock during the night
- keep the bedroom just for sleep and sex.

This advice can and should be modified when necessary. For instance, a nap the day of a very important evening event can make all the difference. And an occasional lie-in can save the weekend for both herself and her partner. Besides, being too rigid with advice can cost you your patient's trust.

As you talk to Sophie, you realize she has a very sedentary lifestyle. Working from home, she doesn't have much demarcation between work and leisure, and when you explore a bit further you find out she often sits in bed with her laptop over emails or unfinished work.

What can you usefully suggest to her? Write down at least four recommendations.

- Take regular **exercise**.
- Cut out the last cup of **tea**, and some of the **coffee**.
- Reduce her **alcohol** consumption.
- Consider **formal working hours**, even at home.

Sophie is pleased to have been given advice and is hopeful that it will help.

She returns a few weeks later, having reduced her alcohol and caffeine intake. She goes swimming a couple of times a week, and aims to take a walk after her evening meal. Now she leaves her mobile and her laptop in the living room at night. She is still a bit of a worrier about work, but her sleeping is a slightly better, with the exception of Sunday nights when she frets about the week ahead.

Resources
CKS/NICE Insomnia.
  http://cks.nice.org.uk/insomnia
DVLA: driver's medical enquiries information.
  https://www.gov.uk/dvla-medical-enquiries

CASE

17

My eye hurts

Rona McIver, age 32 years
Teacher
PMH: sciatica 18/12 ago; TOP age 17; labyrinthitis
Medication: oral contraceptive pill

Rona McIver moved to the area recently to live with her partner, and this is her first visit to your practice apart from her new patient check. Today she has a one-day history of left eye pain, worse on movement. There is no redness, itching or discharge, and no history of trauma. She says her vision is 'a wee bit weird' and that colours are 'blurry'. She has no previous eye symptoms and does not wear contact lenses. She feels well, though her new teaching job is tiring.

What should you do?

Fully examine both eyes, including visual **acuity**, **colour** vision, **fundoscopy**, **EOM** and pupil reactions.

Rona's vision is 6/6 in both eyes, and you cannot find Ishihara colour plates. Both eyes are quiet, the pupils equal and the fundi normal. Eye movements are normal if uncomfortable.

The right pupil responds to light and accommodation but does not constrict when you shine your light in the left eye. The left pupil does not respond to light, but does show consensual constriction.

What does this mean?

She has a left **afferent pupillary defect**. The swinging light test would show the so-called Marcus Gunn pupil. The defect is clear in Rona's case, but in some patients both eyes are affected or there are complicating factors (see Resources).

► An afferent pupillary defect usually signifies a problem of the optic nerve. It occurs in various conditions including:

- acute glaucoma
- trauma
- tumours
- optic neuritis.

Features of optic neuritis

- Ocular/retrobulbar pain, especially on movement.
- Some visual impairment which can be mild or severe.
- Impaired colour vision.

What should you do?

You should refer Rona to the urgent eye clinic to be seen the same day. Rona takes it in her stride when you say you're not sure what's going on, but you'd like a specialist opinion.

You later learn that Rona was diagnosed with optic neuritis and is now better. The letter mentions possible neurological referral but nothing has been arranged.

What should you do?

(a) Refer Rona now without seeing her?
(b) Review Rona first then refer her?
(c) Leave things for now as Rona is now better?
Although optic neuritis can be an isolated event, NICE guidance recommends **neurological referral for every confirmed case**. So (b) is the best course of action.

- NICE also advises GPs to instigate **blood tests to rule out other diagnoses** before referral: FBC, ESR and/or CRP, LFTs, U&E and creatinine, calcium, glucose, TFTs, serum B12 and HIV serology. You could also consider serology for syphilis.

You have not yet done a neurological **examination**.

You should also **discuss the referral** with Rona.

Rona returns to see you. She feels OK though her job is quite draining. She does not have a neurology appointment.

What in particular should you examine?

- Power in the limbs.
- Sensation if you have time.
- Reflexes: tendon reflexes, plantars and abdominal reflexes.
- Cranial nerves, including the lower cranial nerves to test bulbar function.
- Balance and coordination: Romberg's test, heel–toe walking, finger–nose test.
- Check for nystagmus, which is common in MS.
- Check for Lhermitte's.

The clinical manifestations of MS

Highly varied. Symptoms often evolve over >24 hours, lasting days or weeks before improving. Common features:

- Paraesthesiae (often an early complaint).
- Optic neuritis.
- Other eye symptoms (e.g. diplopia on lateral gaze).
- Spinal cord involvement (e.g. muscle cramping or bladder/bowel disturbance).
- Cerebellar symptoms (dysarthria, clumsiness, tremor).
- Trigeminal neuralgia.
- Facial muscle twitching.
- Fatigue.
- Cognitive problems (e.g. poor concentration, attention span).
- Constitutional symptoms (e.g. fatigue, dizziness).
- Depression (much more common than euphoria).

Tips

- There may be no abnormal findings between relapses.
- In optic neuritis the optic nerve can look normal.
- Abdominal reflexes are usually absent in established MS.

Rona's limb power is normal though the reflexes are a bit brisk. Plantars are downgoing. Her cranial nerves are normal (instead of testing the lower cranial nerves, you ask about swallowing and

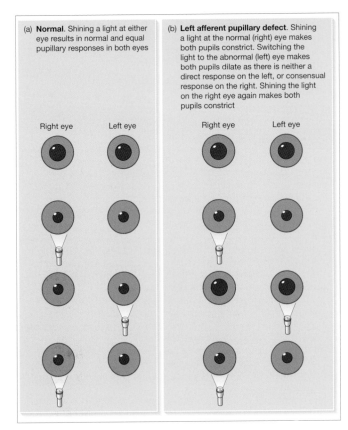

(a) **Normal**. Shining a light at either eye results in normal and equal pupillary responses in both eyes

(b) **Left afferent pupillary defect**. Shining a light at the normal (right) eye makes both pupils constrict. Switching the light to the abnormal (left) eye makes both pupils dilate as there is neither a direct response on the left, or consensual response on the right. Shining the light on the right eye again makes both pupils constrict

Figure 17.1 Pupillary reactions in the swinging light test.

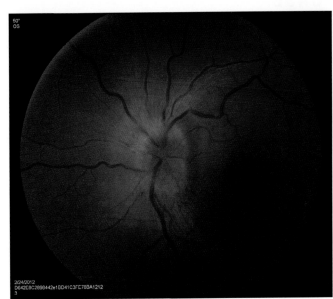

Figure 17.2 Papilloedema.

Source: Olver J et al. (2014) *Ophthalmology at a Glance*, 2nd edn. Reproduced with permission of Jane Olver.

Classification of MS

Overall, MS leads to significant physical disability within 20–25 years in about a third of patients. There are distinct types of disease.

Relapsing–remitting (about 85%)

- Distinct attacks of symptoms which then fade either partially or completely.
- Early therapy gives better outcomes.
- Many with RRMS go on to have secondary progressive MS.

Primary progressive (about 10–15%)

Symptoms in PPMS gradually worsen over time, without sudden relapses.

Progressive–relapsing (rare, <5%)

Progressive worsening from the start, with acute relapses but no remissions.

Benign

Like relapsing remitting, but very mild attacks separated by long periods with no symptoms. Can only be diagnosed with hindsight after 10–15 years.

speaking, and she says it is all 'fine'). Her heel–toe walking is hesitant but all else on your list is normal.

In reviewing her past history, you discover that her sciatica was pins and needles going up the leg. It lasted four weeks and there wasn't any back pain or injury. Her labyrinthitis made her very unsteady and she had time off work. That lasted three weeks. Neither symptom was investigated, according to the notes. It's possible that both episodes were manifestations of MS.

What do you do now?

Refer her to the neurologist as MS is the likely diagnosis here.

You tell Rona that you found nothing obviously wrong, but she needs a blood test and a proper neurology assessment. She does not ask more. Do not tell her that her previous GP may have misdiagnosed her, as you do not have all the details, and cannot be sure she has MS. It is also counterproductive to criticize colleagues. However that should not stop you, if you find it appropriate, from telling Rona that her previous symptoms may turn out to have been significant.

Weeks later, a neurologist's letter tells you Rona has MS.

While MS is incurable, newer biological treatments can reduce the number and severity of attacks. In the more distant future, stem cells may eventually realize their promise too.

GPs can play a large part in managing MS:

- supporting the patient
- helping to modify the factors associated with relapse
- offering symptomatic relief (e.g. for bladder frequency, muscle spasms, pain, depression, fatigue).

Resources

NICE guidance: Multiple sclerosis – management of multiple sclerosis in primary and secondary care.
www.nice.org.uk/guidance/cg186/chapter/1-recommendations#diagnosing-ms-2

Colorblind (includes online Ishihara test with eight plates).
http://colorvisiontesting.com

Broadway DC. How to test for a relative afferent pupillary defect (RAPD). *Community Eye Health Journal* 2012.
www.ncbi.nlm.nih.gov/pmc/articles/PMC3588138/pdf/jceh_25_79-80_058.pdf

GMC guidance: Good medical practice.
http://www.gmc-uk.org/guidance/good_medical_practice.asp

MS Society (charity for patients, families and professionals).
www.mssociety.org.uk/

MS Trust (charity for information, education, research and support).
www.mstrust.org.uk/

CASE

18

I think I should get this prostate test, doctor

Barrington Dixon, age 66 years

Retired

PMH: cataract   Medication: nil

Mr and Mrs Dixon and their family have been registered with the practice for almost 50 years, having been born in Jamaica. Mr Dixon sits down and says, 'I think I should get this prostate test, doctor.'

What should you ask first?

The first thing you should explore is Mr Dixon's reasons for wanting the test. This should be done with a nice open question, such as, 'Tell me why you're thinking about getting the test?'

Mr Dixon goes on to explain that one of his good friends, James, has recently been diagnosed with prostate cancer. James became quite unwell quickly and Mr Dixon understands that the cancer has already spread to his bones. Mr Dixon remembers that an uncle of his back in Jamaica had 'some kind of prostate problem'. Mr Dixon is worried that he could have a silent prostate cancer, and now he and his friends are all thinking about getting the test.

What symptoms should you enquire about?

Ask an open question first, such as, 'Have you noticed any symptoms?'

Lower urinary tract symptoms (LUTS, such as poor stream, nocturia and frequency) can be associated with prostate cancer, but are far more likely to represent benign prostatic hypertrophy.

Specific symptoms that do have an association with prostate cancer and are worth asking about explicitly are:

▶ **bone pain** and ▶ **haematuria**.

Mr Dixon doesn't have any new symptoms. He has been getting up to pass urine in the night two or three times for many years now.

How would you best counsel Mr Dixon about the test?

You should have an open discussion so that Mr Dixon is able to make an **informed decision** about whether or not he should have a PSA test. There are some excellent patient information resources (see Resources) that can be useful in guiding his decision.

The PSA test has significant limitations (see Table 18.1) but it is currently the best test available for identifying a localized prostate cancer. The test does not meet the standards for a population-based screening programme so is currently being offered on an 'as requested' basis.

Mr Dixon, having discussed the above with you, is keen to go ahead and have the PSA test. You offer simple advice on conservative measures that might improve his LUTS (for example, reduced caffeine and alcohol intake), and explore the option of medical treatment for these symptoms. Mr Dixon is not interested in these at the moment.

Are there any practicalities you should advise Mr Dixon about before having the test?

Patient should not have:
- an active UTI
- had a digital rectal examination in the last week
- ejaculated or exercised vigorously in the last 48 hours.

Table 18.1 Potential benefits and limitations of PSA test.

Potential benefits of PSA test
May be reassuring if the test is normal
May lead to detection of cancer before symptoms develop
May lead to detection of cancer at early stage (for example at a curable stage or when treatment could extend life)
Could be repeated in future, allowing monitoring of trend

Limitations of PSA test
It is not diagnostic. Further tests would be required for this (for example transurethral resection of prostate (TURP), which carries its own risks of long-term complications such as incontinence and erectile dysfunction)
It is not specific. Many other conditions increase the PSA level (for example benign prostatic hyperplasia (BPH), urinary tract Infection (UTI) and prostatitis). About two in three men with a raised PSA will not have prostate cancer
Many cases of prostate cancer do not cause an elevation of the PSA. The Prostate Cancer Risk Management Programme quotes data showing that 15% of men with a normal PSA may have prostate cancer (see Resources)
The test may lead to the diagnosis of cancers that may never become apparent or shorten the patient's life

What other test should you offer Mr Dixon?

- Opportunistic screening for **diabetes** may also be appropriate. This patient is at high risk given his age and ethnicity (Afro-Caribbean), so he should have an Hba1c blood test.
- You may also want to consider an opportunistic **lipid profile**.
- As he has not attended for some time, you should also check his **blood pressure**.

Mr Dixon is very happy to go ahead and have both a diabetes screen and a lipid profile. You check his blood pressure and it is 122/62.

Mr Dixon's blood tests return the following week (Table 18.2).

Table 18.2 Mr Dixon's blood test results.

Parameter	Result
PSA	2.04 ng/mL
Hba1c	44 mmol/mol (6.2%)
Total cholesterol	4.8 mmol/L

Mr Dixon's PSA is reassuringly normal, but what does he have?

Mr Dixon's Hba1c is indicative of 'pre-diabetes' (Hba1c 42–47 mmol/mol or 6.0–6.4% inclusive). He would benefit from referral to a diabetes education programme. This will help him know how to prevent this from progressing to diabetes. His Hba1c should be rechecked in 6 months' time.

You discuss this with Mr Dixon and he is glad to know that his PSA is normal. He closes by saying that maybe James' illness was a wake-up call. He has plans to get back to fitness and start swimming again.

Resources

Prostate Cancer Risk Management Programme – Information for Primary Care.

http://www.cancerscreening.nhs.uk/prostate/prostate-booklet-text.pdf

General Practice Cases at a Glance, First Edition. Carol Cooper and Martin L Block. © 2017 John Wiley & Sons, Ltd. Published 2017 by John Wiley & Sons, Ltd.

CASE
19 I can't live with this pain much longer

Susan Barnes, age 58 years
Housewife
PMH: hysterectomy; shoulder injury
Medication: co-codamol, simvastatin

Mrs Barnes is new to the practice. She is holding her right wrist as she tells you the pain is unbearable. It started shortly after she injured her arm a year ago, and has been there for nearly 10 months.

Sometimes it feels like it's all the way down the arm and into the hand, but usually it's the wrist and hand, like today, and it stops her sleeping. She saw an orthopaedic surgeon for the pain twice but nothing was done for her. Nothing seems to make it better, and she can't always predict what will make it worse.

Mrs Barnes lives with her newly retired husband and no longer works. She clearly has chronic pain (pain that has persisted more than 12 weeks and is out of keeping with the original trigger).

What useful questions would you ask? Write down at least seven.

- 'Are you **right**- or **left-handed**?' This is a basic question whenever a patient has upper limb symptoms.
- 'Tell me **more about the pain**.' It may be crushing, dull, burning, shooting, tingling, like an electric shock, numb, prickling or itching.
- 'Do you get **pins and needles**?' This can be a sign of neuropathic pain.
- 'On a **scale of 0–10**, how would you score this pain?' It's sometimes useful to compare it with previous pain, e.g. labour.
- 'What does it **stop you doing**?' Assessment of function is vital.
- 'How much does it **get you down**?' is one way of opening a discussion about mood. As she says she can't live with this pain, it's wise to assess her mental state.
- ▶ 'Have you **lost weight**?' Ask also about other red flags such as ▶ constant **unremitting pain** and ▶ **fever** or **sweating**, and ask about any PMH of **cancer**.
- What are her **ICE**? You could ask her what she's hoping for, and why she came now.

Mrs Barnes is nearly in tears as she tells you it's often a score of 7–9, depending on the day. The pain is burning, sometimes tight, and she gets pins and needles. It's not there all the time and she has no systemic symptoms.

She's right-handed so she has to use a mouse with her left hand. She had a part-time job in a school but she gave that up anyway when she moved. She wouldn't be able to work now. She can hardly keep up with housework. She's beginning to think the pain can't be cured, but her daughter is getting married in six weeks and she'd like to feel better.

Chronic pain is a common condition, affecting around 15% of the population. Some 25% of those diagnosed lose their jobs. About 70% of those living with chronic pain are under 60. The majority is managed in primary care, and, even when secondary care is involved, the GP may need to look after the patient between pain clinic appointments.

Chronic pain isn't just acute pain that has stayed too long. Changes occur in the brain and spinal cord, so the pain is perceived differently. There's often loss of function, psychological distress or depression, and behavioural change. It's a complex bio-psycho-social condition.

> **Tip**
> A word about terminology: while 'chronic pain' is the term doctors most often use, 'persistent pain' is equally accurate. The two phrases are interchangeable, but 'persistent pain' is less dispiriting for patients to hear.

Some causes of persistent pain

Common
- Low back pain.
- Degenerative joint disease.
- Myofascial pain syndromes (e.g. fibromyalgia, RSI).

Other
- Pelvic pain.
- Abdominal pain (e.g. gall bladder disease).
- Post-op pain.
- Post-herpetic pain.
- Diabetic neuropathy.
- Other types of neuropathy.
- Chronic headaches.
- Stroke.
- MS.
- Trigeminal neuralgia.
- Complex regional pain syndrome (CPRS) – also known as Sudeck's atrophy, shoulder–hand syndrome, reflex sympathetic dystrophy.

Any system of the body can give rise to chronic pain.

Does she have neuropathic pain?

She probably does. Neuropathic pain develops from damage to or dysfunction of the nervous system. Pain can be intermittent or constant.

- The pain is either **shooting**, **stabbing**, like an electric shock, **burning**, **tingling**, tight, numb, prickling or itching.
- **Allodynia** – pain is triggered by light touch or some other stimulus that isn't normally painful.
- **Hyperalgesia** – increased response to a painful stimulus.

The significance is that the treatment of neuropathic pain is different, but not everyone has all the typical symptoms.

You examine Mrs Barnes. Her right wrist and hand look normal. Light touch is painful, as is vibration, making it hard to assess sensation. Shoulder, elbow and wrist movements are full, but her grip strength is reduced on the right. Neck movements are also normal.

Does she have complex regional pain syndrome?

Probably not, but it is something you should think of, especially with chronic upper limb pain. There are diagnostic criteria, as well as specialized treatments including physiotherapy, so everyone with CRPS should be referred to an appropriate secondary care specialist.

CRPS

Chronic condition of unknown cause, with limb pain and dysfunction within the motor, sensory and autonomic nervous systems. Usually post-traumatic (e.g. after fractured radius or shoulder injury) but 10% are spontaneous. Can occur in children.

Typical features
- pain disproportionate to that expected
- abnormal swelling
- abnormal colour (e.g. red, mottled or cyanosed, or a mixture)
- abnormal temperature
- abnormal sweating
- motor dysfunction (e.g. clumsiness)
- abnormal skin or nail appearance
- limb may feel 'as if doesn't belong' to the patient.

Outlook is variable, with long-term pain and work problems in about 50%.

What are you going to do now for Mrs Barnes?

Persistent pain is often a worsening cycle, with many aspects (Figure 19.1). Mrs Barnes needs a holistic approach.
- Supported self-management: use recommended self-help resources (e.g. Pain Toolkit) at any stage as needed.

- Biological (i.e. drug) therapy: see box for options.
- Psychosocial therapy: assess depressive symptoms. CBT or counselling may help chronic pain, or refer to a pain clinic.
- Physical therapy: exercise is recommended for all chronic pain patients. They may also benefit from specific physiotherapy.

Tip
Don't feel under pressure to cover everything in this consultation. Chronic pain takes time to assess and to manage.

Mrs Barnes appears tired but not low or depressed and has no suicidal ideation. She has already had a range of NSAIDs as well as co-codamol, but has not tried tricyclics or anti-epileptics. You discuss the options. As her pain sounds neuropathic, you begin amitriptyline 25 mg nightly increasing to bd, with co-dydramol to take as and when needed (see box for other choices). This may help her sleep as well.

Mrs Barnes may also benefit from a referral to physiotherapy and/or to local counselling services. If your efforts to manage her in primary care are not successful, another option would be referral to the pain clinic. Remember that even if you refer her today, it will be some time before she is seen.

It's important for chronic pain patients to be believed. Try something like, 'You must find this very difficult', or, 'The pain seems very bad.' CBT can usefully reframe the patient's thinking, but it won't make the pain disappear. There is a CNS element, so you could explain there are brain changes when people have to live

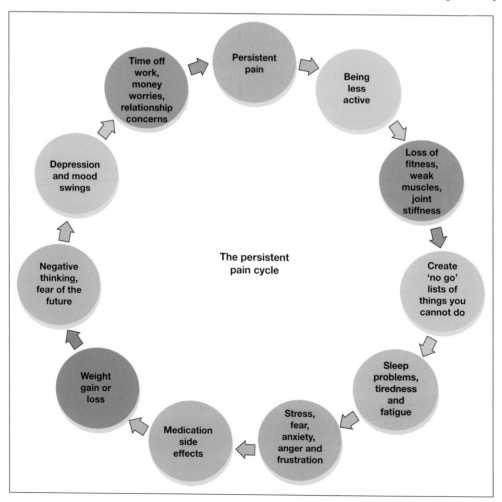

Figure 19.1 The persistent pain cycle.

Source: Reproduced with permission of www.paintoolkit.org.

Drugs for chronic pain

Worth using, but only a third of patients get 50% reduction of pain.

Non-opioid

- NSAIDs especially for low back pain (consider GI/CVS risks).
- Paracetamol 1–4 g daily alone or with NSAIDs.
- Topical NSAIDs for MSK conditions, especially if cannot tolerate oral NSAIDs.
- Consider topical capsaicin patches for peripheral neuropathic pain if other treatments don't help.
- Consider topical rubefacients for MSK pain if other treatments don't help.
- Consider topical lidocaine for post-herpetic pain if other treatments don't help.

Opioids

- Carefully assess risk factors for opioid misuse.
- Consider for chronic low back pain or osteoarthritis – only continue if there is continued pain relief.
- Always advise about common side effects, and review regularly.
- Can be used as additional medication on bad days.
- Refer if concerns about dose escalation.

Anti-epileptics

Useful for neuropathic and myofascial pain.
- Gabapentin or pregabalin for neuropathic pain.
- Pregabalin for fibromyalgia.
- Carbamazepine for trigeminal/other neuropathic pain.

Antidepressants

- Tricyclic antidepressants (e.g. amitriptyline 25–125 mg daily) for neuropathic pain or fibromyalgia.
- Consider fluoxetine or duloxetine for fibromyalgia.
- Consider duloxetine for diabetic neuropathic pain if other agents fail.

Antidepressants may be needed for their antidepressant action also.

For neuropathic pain (except trigeminal neuralgia)

Offer a choice of amitriptyline, duloxetine, gabapentin or pregabalin as initial therapy.

with pain: 'The pain isn't in your mind, but it is in the head as much as in the arm.'

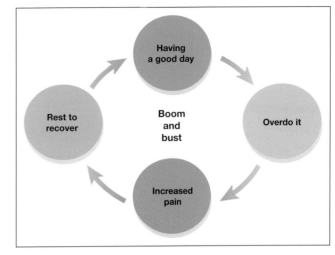

Figure 19.2 Boom and bust cycle.
Source: Reproduced with permission of www.paintoolkit.org.

She needs help with her daily life too. Could her husband do more housework? Can she pace herself, especially in the run-up to her daughter's wedding when she probably has a lot to do? Typically chronic pain patients go through 'boom and bust' behaviour (Figure 19.2). Frustration over limitations leads to overactivity, then a flare of pain, followed by prolonged immobility to compensate, and inevitable worsening, which leads to increased frustration.

Finally remember to arrange to see her again to explore all you have not been able to do today, and to see how she is doing. Given her daughter's imminent wedding, an appointment next week or the week after might be suitable.

Resources

SIGN guideline 136 Management of chronic pain.
    www.sign.ac.uk/pdf/SIGN136.pdf
CKS/NICE Neuropathic pain – drug treatment.
    cks.nice.org.uk/neuropathic-pain-drug-treatment#!
    backgroundsub
Royal College of Physicians: Complex regional pain syndrome.
    www.rcplondon.ac.uk/sites/default/files/documents/complex-
    regional-pain-full-guideline.pdf
Pain Toolkit.
    www.paintoolkit.org/ (for patients)
    http://www.paintoolkit.org/resources/healthcare-professionals
    (for healthcare professionals)

CASE

20

I've got a red eye

Peter Borowicz, age 36 years

IT engineer

PMH: nil of note

Medication: nil

Mr Borowicz has booked into an early morning emergency appointment. As he sits down, you see he has an obvious red eye. You ask him what you can do for him today, and he laughs as he says 'I don't know if you've noticed, but my eye is red.' He tells you that he woke up yesterday and his eye was red and sticky. He is concerned about what might be going on. He never normally gets ill and has never had any eye problems before.

What are the possible red flags that might indicate a serious cause? Write down at least four.

The presence of any of the features in the box below could suggest a serious cause for his red eye. Patients with these should be seen urgently, on the same day, in an acute eye unit. You should ask specifically about each of these.

Red eye – the red flags

- ► Moderate or severe eye pain.
- ► Moderate or severe photophobia.
- ► Marked redness of one eye.
- ► Decrease in visual acuity.
- ► Possible penetrating injury.

Cause	Symptoms and signs	Management
(a) Infective conjunctivitis	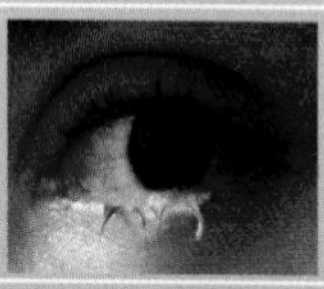 Red conjunctiva Can be sticky in the morning Unilateral or bilateral Not especially painful and acuity unaffected	Regular washes Consider antibiotic drops
(b) Allergic conjunctivitis	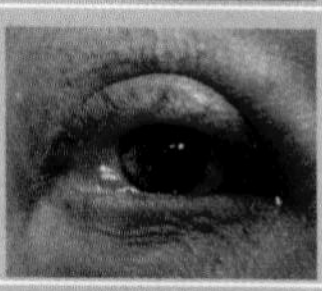 Itchy and a little swollen Bilaterally engorged conjunctiva Watery Painless, and acuity unaffected	Avoid allergen Avoid rubbing eye Antihistamines (oral or topical) Topical sodium cromoglycate
(c) Blepharitis	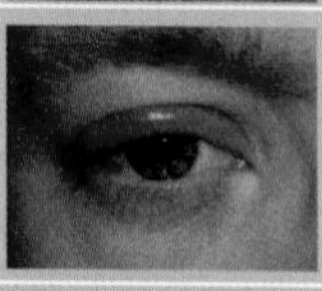 Sticky and sometimes flaky eyelids Not painful and acuity unaffected	Eyelid hygiene
(d) Acute glaucoma	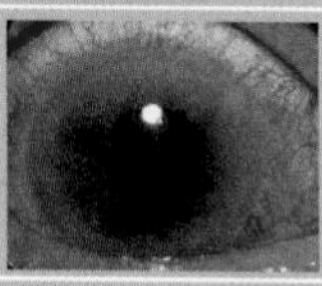 Acutely very painful red eye Visual disturbance Feels unwell Fixed dilated pupil	Emergency to eye casualty
(e) Uveitis	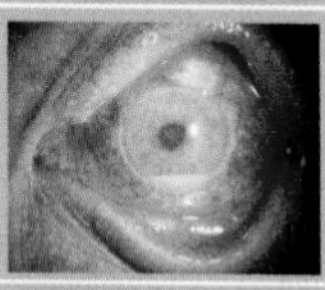 Painful red eye Vision may be impaired Photophobia	Refer to eye casualty for further assessment
(f) Scleritis	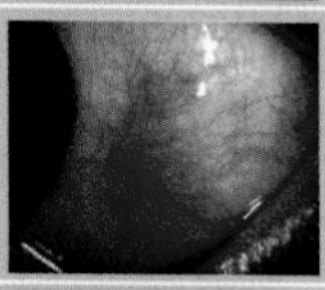 Red painful focally engorged conjunctiva	Refer to eye casualty for further assessment
(g) Subconjunctival haemorrhage	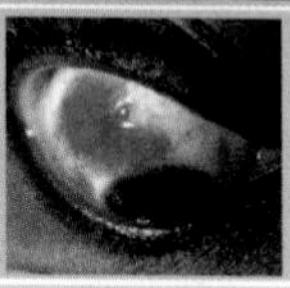 Appearance of burst blood vessel in eye Not painful and acuity unaffected	Check BP Resolves spontaneously over 2–3 weeks

Figure 20.1 Causes of acute red eye.

Source: (a) Tanalai. https://commons.wikimedia.org/wiki/File:Swollen_eye_with_conjunctivitis.jpg. Used under CCA 3.0; (b) James Heilman, MD. https://commons.wikimedia.org/wiki/File:Allergicconjunctivitis.jpg. Used under CCA-SA 4.0; (c) clubtable. https://commons.wikimedia.org/wiki/File:Blepharitis.JPG. Public domain; (d) Jonathan Trobe, M.D. https://commons.wikimedia.org/wiki/File:Acute_Angle_Closure-glaucoma.jpg. Used under CCA 3.0; (e) EyeMD. https://commons.wikimedia.org/wiki/File:Hypopyon.jpg. Used under CCA SA 2.5; (f) Kribz. https://commons.wikimedia.org/wiki/File:Scleritis.png. Used under CCA-SA 3.0; (g) Olver J et al. (2014) *Ophthalmology at a Glance*, 2nd edn. Reproduced with permission of Jane Olver.

Aside from red flags, what else would you like to ask about?

Find out about any other associated symptoms.

- 'Is it itchy?' Itch suggests allergy.
- 'Is there any discharge?' This can occur with infection.
- 'Any recent contact with anyone with similar symptoms?'
- 'Do you wear contact lenses?' Infection in contact lens wearers can be very serious, e.g. acanthamoeba keratitis.

Mr Borowicz tells you that his eye is not painful, but it does feel a little gritty. Fortunately the light is not a problem (he works as an IT engineer) and, apart from a little watering, his vision has been unaffected. He certainly cannot recall any recent penetrating injury. The eye is not itchy but there is some discharge. This is worse in the mornings and he has to clean his eye to remove this when he wakes up.

Describe your examination

You should examine **both eyes**, checking both conjunctivae, pupils and eyelids. If there is any suggestion of a decrease in acuity you should formally assess acuity using a **Snellen chart**.

Mr Borowicz has a mild to moderately engorged conjunctiva in his right eye. There is some mild yellowish discharge. His pupils are unaffected. His left eye is normal. You decide to check his acuity, which is 6/9 bilaterally (uncorrected).

What is the most likely diagnosis?

The most likely diagnosis is infective conjunctivitis.

How should you treat infective conjunctivitis?

In most cases, infective conjunctivitis is a self-limiting illness that resolves without treatment in 1–2 weeks. During this time you should advise conservative management:

- clean away secretions regularly
- wash hands regularly
- over-the-counter lubricant eye drops will ease irritation.

Consider a topical antibiotic (e.g. chloramphenicol eye drops) if symptoms are more significant, or fail to resolve. Schools may not allow a child to return unless treatment is started, which may influence your management.

You explain to Mr Borowicz that the condition is likely to be self-limiting and not anything dangerous. He is happy with this, and is glad that he doesn't need to use eye drops. He asks you how easy it is to spread it to his wife and children, so you advise him on the importance of regular hand washing and of not sharing towels and pillows.

What safety net should you put in place?

A good safety net is clear and specific. Mr Borowicz needs to know the specific things that would make it necessary for him to return to the GP.

- Development of red flag symptoms:

  ▶ pain

  ▶ photophobia

  ▶ loss of acuity

  ▶ significant increase in redness.

- Persistence of symptoms (beyond two weeks).

You give Mr Borowicz this information and he leaves your room, heading off to work.

Resources

CKS/NICE Red eye.
   http://cks.nice.org.uk/red-eye

CASE
21   I'm fed up with my spots

Lucy Cartwright, age 15 years
Lives at home with parents and younger brother James
PMH: nil of note
Medication: nil

Lucy Cartwright is booked in to see you in your afternoon surgery. She attends today with someone else around her age.

You welcome Lucy into your room. What else should you do?

You should also find out who else has come down with her today. In this case you find out that Lucy is accompanied by Megan, who is a friend from school. Lucy tells you that her mum can't come down today because she is collecting James from school. You ask Lucy what you can do for her today.

Lucy tells you that she is fed up with her spots. You give her some time to talk and she tells you more. She has had spots for a couple of years. She really hates them. They started out as being quite small, but now she gets some larger spots that last for longer. She is really fed up with them and is desperate for them to go away. At this point Lucy looks down to the ground, looking sad, whilst Megan gives her a kind, reassuring look.

Is Lucy giving you any cues that you could respond to?

Lucy has hinted that she is quite distressed by her spots. This is something you could pick up and explore further. A good way of doing this is to pick up something she has said and to reflect it back.

Cues – verbal and non-verbal

In the consultation, keep your eyes open to **cues**.

A cue is a hint that the patient is giving you about an area that you may benefit from exploring further. This may tell you more about areas such as what the patient is worried about, or the impact the condition is having.

Following cues often gives you really interesting and useful information.

Cues can be **verbal** or **non-verbal**. In this case Lucy has given out some verbal cues, she is 'fed up' with her spots, she 'really hates them' and she is 'desperate for them to go away'. She has also given a non-verbal cue, with her sad look to the ground.

If you **listen** to and **observe** your patient attentively, you will notice the cues.

Think of a way that you might use reflection here.

One way would be to say, 'You sound quite fed up with your spots.'

Following this, Lucy goes into a little more detail. She feels ashamed and embarrassed and wishes every day that they will just go away. She has the worst spots of anyone in her class, and she is very conscious of this.

What other areas should you cover? Think of three.

• What has she tried already? You should check and find out what **treatments** (if any) Lucy has tried.
• What **areas** are affected? Acne commonly appears on the back or the chest as well as the face.
• Is there any variation with her **menstrual cycle**? Some women experience a flare-up around the time of menstruation. Are there any features to suggest **PCOS** (e.g. irregular periods, hirsutism)? This can be a cause of acne.

Lucy has tried various over-the-counter remedies and medicated soaps. She has also tried rubbing TCP into her spots, but this only made matters worse. She tells you that it is just her face that is affected. Her skin is bad throughout the month. Lucy has not noticed any variation with her periods.

What examination should you do?

You should examine the affected area(s). In this case you examine Lucy's face. You should assess the distribution of the spots, the type of spots and if there is any scarring.

Lucy has a collection of acne spots, with scattered blackheads on her forehead and around her cheeks and three or four inflamed whiteheads on her forehead. This is no scarring.

At this point in the consultation you should explain the diagnosis.

How would you do this?

Lucy has a diagnosis of acne. You should offer a clear, concise explanation in non-medical jargon, such as, 'The spots you have are caused by acne. The pores in your skin become blocked and this in turn can get infected causing the spots.' Your explanation should always feel comfortable for you. A **patient information leaflet** would be helpful here. There are lots of useful resources online, such as the patient.co.uk information leaflets that explain the causes and treatment of acne.

Acne – myth busters

• Acne is not caused by poor hygiene. Excessive washing may make it worse.
• Acne is not caused by stress.
• Acne is not contagious.
• Drinking lots of water does not help.
• Sunbathing or sunbeds do not help.

What should guide your decision to treat?

Your management should be guided by the severity of the acne and the distressed caused. Lucy has moderate acne and it is causing significant distress. It definitely warrants treatment. The aim of treatment is to minimize the number of spots as much as possible and to prevent scarring.

What treatment options should you consider? Think of three.

There are several options open to you, and these are outlined in Table 21.1.

General Practice Cases at a Glance, First Edition. Carol Cooper and Martin L Block. © 2017 John Wiley & Sons, Ltd. Published 2017 by John Wiley & Sons, Ltd.

Table 21.1 Treatment of acne.

Type of treatment	Examples
Topical preparations	Benzoyl peroxide Topical retinoids Topical antibiotics Azelaic acid
Oral antibiotics	Tetracyclines (such as oxytetracycline, doxycycline and lymecycline) Not to be taken if planning to become pregnant
Combined oral contraceptive	Especially helpful if the acne is affected by the menstrual cycle
Oral retinoids	Roaccutane This can currently only be prescribed in a specialist setting

You spend some time go through the treatment options with Lucy, backed up by a patient information leaflet that helpfully goes through all the different options with you. Lucy is very engaged with this and is very keen to try something that will get rid of the spots as soon as possible. She is reluctant to consider going on to the Pill, and she is also worried about what her mother will think. She is keen to try a cream alongside an antibiotic tablet as she is hopeful that this will give her the best chance of getting rid of her spots.

You and Lucy decide on a treatment regime of topical benzoyl peroxide and oral oxytetracycline. You give Lucy the prescription and warn her it may take 6–8 weeks to see any improvement. You advise her to make a follow-up appointment to see you in three months' time. She is grateful to you for taking the problem seriously.

A final word on competence

Lucy is 15 and is legally defined as a child. Ideally she ought to be seen with a parent. This case should make you think about whether or not to treat a child without the presence of a parent. To help guide you, consider whether a child is 'Gillick competent':

'…it is not enough that she should understand the nature of the advice which is being given: she must also have a sufficient maturity to understand what is involved.' (from NSPCC commentary on Gillick Competence)

Lucy has the maturity to understand her condition and treatment, and is therefore competent to make an autonomous decision about her health.

Resources

Patient information on acne.
>   http://www.patient.co.uk/health/acne

Gillick competency.
>   http://www.nspcc.org.uk/preventing-abuse/child-protection-system/legal-definition-child-rights-law/gillick-competency-fraser-guidelines/

You may also like to try Case 39: 'I don't want to have my period when I'm on holiday'.

CASE

22 I've come for the results of my blood tests

Derek Connor, age 57 years

Restaurant owner

PMH: nil of note

Medication: nil

Ex-smoker

Mr Connor has recently attended for an NHS Health Check with the practice healthcare assistant, Daisy. Looking down his records it's clear that Mr Connor rarely attends the surgery. Looking at Daisy's notes from his last consultation you see:

- blood pressure 133/71
- urine dipstick NAD
- BMI 29.8.

Daisy has also noted that Mr Connor has a family history of type 2 diabetes (both older brothers) and that he is from a Black British (Afro-Caribbean) background. She also notes that he is feeling well.

It appears that one of your colleagues, having seen Mr Connor's blood results, wrote to him, requesting that he repeat one of the tests and to book in to see the doctor to discuss the results.

Mr Connor's first words to you today are, 'I've come for the results of my blood tests.'

You look at these results on the system (Table 22.1).

What is the diagnosis?

Mr Connor has type 2 diabetes.

What factors support the diagnosis of type 2 over type 1 diabetes? Name three.

- **Age**: onset of type 1 is much more common in younger patients.
- **Urinalysis**: no ketones or glucose on first presentation.
- **Absence of symptoms**: type 1 tends to be symptomatic at first presentation (and patient is often quite unwell), while type 2 can be symptomatic or asymptomatic.

What is your first priority for this consultation?

The first and **most important** priority is that Mr Connor understands his new diagnosis of diabetes. There are lots of really helpful resources to help you here, including patient information leaflets and websites such as Diabetes UK (www.diabetes.org.uk).

How would you explain this new diagnosis? Try practising your wording.

As always, be clear and concise. Try something like, 'Diabetes is a condition in which the body is unable to control the level of sugar in the blood. The sugar level is usually under the control of a hormone called insulin. In diabetes, either the body produces less insulin, or the insulin produced is not able to work properly. This causes the sugar level to rise.'

It is always worth checking now that your patient has understood your diagnosis, allowing him time to ask any questions, and giving him space to discuss further. Do not rush here.

Mr Connor tells you that his older brothers both have diabetes so he is quite familiar with it. He is though very disappointed and a little upset to be given this diagnosis. One of his brothers (the eldest, Roy) is on insulin. Mr Connor is very keen to avoid this. Roy also has a 'weak kidney' and is 'half blind' due to his diabetes. The middle brother Courtney seems OK, he is just on tablet medication. Mr Connor asks you if he needs to start on insulin.

Does Mr Connor need to start insulin now?

No. There are other treatments that should be used as first line.

Before going into detail about the treatments, what should you do first?

You should describe **why** you are treating Mr Connor's diabetes. After all, Mr Connor doesn't have any symptoms right now.

Think now of how you would explain this to Mr Connor.

As before, keep this clear and concise. An example could be, 'We know that people who have diabetes have a higher risk of developing complications in the body's organs, such as the heart, the brain, the eyes and the kidneys. We also know that if we control the blood sugar, blood pressure and cholesterol well, and if you maintain a healthy lifestyle, especially not smoking but also taking regular exercise and eating well, then you can really reduce the risk of complications.' Again, using patient information resources and Diabetes UK's website is useful to illustrate this. It is vital that Mr Connor understands that it's not just about bringing the sugar down. There are lots of other things that are important here.

There is a great deal for the patient to take in. All newly diagnosed diabetics should be referred on to a diabetes education course, such as the DESMOND course. You should refer Mr Connor to this, or a local equivalent.

Mr Connor says this makes sense, and again refers back to Roy's problems with his kidneys and eyes. He asks you if this was because his sugar levels were too high. As there is so much to cover in a new diagnosis of diabetes, Mr Connor may need several appointments with you or the practice nurse initially. There is a good case for all new diabetic patients to be given a 20–30-minute consultation at initial diagnosis.

What are the specific treatment targets for Mr Connor? Name three.

There are several targets to consider (Table 22.2). All of them have an impact on long-term risk of complications.

Table 22.1 Mr Connor's blood test results.

Test 1	
Hba1c	62 mmol/mol (7.8%)
Total cholesterol	5.6 mmol/L
LDL cholesterol	4.1 mmol/L
HDL cholesterol	1.5 mmol/L
U+Es	Normal
Test 2 (2 weeks later)	
Hba1c	61 mmol/mol (7.7%)

General Practice Cases at a Glance, First Edition. Carol Cooper and Martin L Block. © 2017 John Wiley & Sons, Ltd. Published 2017 by John Wiley & Sons, Ltd.

Table 22.2 Targets in type 2 diabetes.

Blood pressure	140/80 130/80 if end-organ damage
Hba1c	If on diet alone or one medication 48 mmol/mol (6.5%) If requiring more intensive treatment 59 mmol/mol (7.5%)
Cholesterol	Total cholesterol: 4.0 mmol/L Most people with type 2 diabetes should be on a statin
Smoking	Non smoking
Diet and lifestyle	Encourage regular exercise Encourage weight loss if overweight

What are your immediate treatment goals for Mr Connor? Write down at least four.

It is vitally important for Mr Connor to have ownership of his treatment goals. The following are the areas that you should advise him to target.

• **Bring down Hba1c.** This may be achieved through diet and exercise. Another option would be to bring in a medication. The first-line drug is metformin, the second-line is gliclazide. Insulin can be considered next.

• **Bring down cholesterol.** Mr Connor should start a statin, such as atorvastatin 40 mg.

• **Maintain good blood pressure.** Mr Connor's blood pressure is fortunately quite good at the moment.

• **Continue to not smoke.** Mr Connor quit smoking almost 10 years ago now, and certainly has no intention to start again.

• **Exercise regularly.** You should advise Mr Connor of the health benefits of exercising for 30–60 minutes four times a week.

Mr Connor is happy to start taking a statin, but is keen to do all he can naturally to being his sugar down. He is going to join the local gym and cut out the cakes, biscuits and Lucozade. You make a plan to reassess his Hba1c in 3–4 months, to see what kind of impact this makes. Again it's really important to go with the patient's motivation here.

As well as working towards the targets, what is the other main part of long-term management?

This is monitoring for **complications**. This is done at diagnosis and at annual review, typically with the practice nurse.

How in practice can you do this? Write down four examples.

• Eyes: annual diabetic eye screening, done through local eye clinic.

• Kidneys: annual blood test (U+E) and urine sample for albumin:creatinine ration (ACR).

• Feet: annual review with nurse, assessing pulses and signs of peripheral neuropathy.

• Erectile dysfunction: ask directly at annual review.

You discuss the above with Mr Connor. He reports no erectile dysfunction at present. You advise Mr Connor to book in to see the nurse in a couple of weeks for a diabetes review, where she will go through the above and address any questions Mr Connor has.

Mr Connor thanks you for taking the time to explain everything clearly. He now feels he has a good understanding of what is going on and what he needs to do. He is looking forward to the diabetes education course and tells you with some certainty, 'You're going to see a different man by the end of the summer.'

Resources

CKS/NICE Type 2 diabetes.
  http://cks.nice.org.uk/diabetes-type-2
Diabetes UK.
  http://www.diabetes.org.uk/
You may also like to try Case 42: 'The nurse did my diabetes check last week. I'm here for the results'.

CASE

23 I'd like to talk to you about HRT

Elizabeth Fraser, age 64 years

Part-time librarian

PMH: two recent UTIs; appendicectomy; breast lump age 40 (benign); back pain – epidural injection

Medication: nil

You have known Mrs Fraser since her husband died suddenly nine years ago. She consults infrequently, though did have a recent UTI. Today she's asking about HRT, which she has never had before. Her menopause was at age 49.

It's unusual for someone so many years post-menopausal to suddenly become interested in HRT, so you try to find out more. She tells you shyly that there is a new man in her life, and 'intimate things' are difficult.

What do you need to establish first?

• **Clarify** what her symptoms are. Is it primarily dryness, or is there persistent dyspareunia (either deep or superficial)?
• Does she have **bladder symptoms**? She consulted for UTI recently; did she think the episodes were related to sex?
• Talking openly without embarrassment should help Mrs Fraser overcome her reticence. Use neutral but exact words (vagina, penetration, passing urine – or passing water) to avoid misunderstandings.

She says her sex drive is normal. Penetration does not hurt as such, but she feels very dry. She has tried K-Y Jelly which did not help much. There is no bleeding. The last UTI did occur after sex.

There are other lubricants on the market. Do you prescribe one now?

You could, though you still need to discuss HRT. Vaginal oestrogens may be more effective than a lubricant and would help symptoms from bladder atrophy as well.

Current guidelines do not in general recommend starting HRT beyond the age of 60, but every woman needs to be considered individually.

Benefits of HRT

• Fewer hot flushes, night sweats (important to menopausal women).
• Fewer aches and pains, better sleep, improved mood possibly (again, not relevant here).
• Relieves symptoms of vaginal atrophy (at almost any age).
• Reduces bladder and urethral atrophy.
• Preserves bone density, hence reduced risk of osteoporosis in spine and hip.
• Reduced cardiovascular risk BUT it is likely to increase the risk in women over 60.
• Possibly: reduced risk of colorectal cancer.

Risks of HRT

• Venous thromboembolic disease is doubled or trebled, especially with combined HRT (but transdermal HRT may not carry the same risk).
• Increased risk of coronary heart disease (in over-60s).
• More likely to develop ischaemic stroke (not with transdermal HRT). This is a dose-related effect.
• Increased risk of breast cancer, though absolute risk is small (1 extra case per 1000 women), and oestrogen-only HRT may not have this effect.
• Increased risk of endometrial cancer with oestrogen-only HRT.
• Possibly: increased risk of ovarian cancer.

What are the important common contraindications to systemic HRT? Write down four. You will find more in your BNF.

► Personal history of breast cancer.
► Personal history of oestrogen-dependent cancer.
► Active or recent cardiovascular disease (angina or MI).
► Venous thromboembolism, especially if recurrent (one-off DVT and on anticoagulants may not contraindicate).
► Thrombophilic disorder (e.g. antiphospholipid syndrome).
► Undiagnosed vaginal bleeding.

While you are thinking things through, Mrs Fraser tells you that her mother and one aunt had severe osteoporosis. She has no sisters, and there are no males with osteoporosis in the family.

What should you do now?

Assess her risk of osteoporosis.

Mrs Fraser weighs 63 kg and is 1.68 m tall. She drinks less than 3 units of alcohol/day and doesn't smoke. The FRAX tool for fracture risk assessment (see Resources) is best used with a bone density measurement, but can be used without one. You find that her risk of osteoporosis is borderline.

Now what do you do?

(a) Prescribe systemic HRT.
(b) Give her lifestyle advice on preventing osteoporosis.
(c) Prescribe topical HRT.
(d) Request bone densitometry (DEXA).
(e) Or something else.

You should give her lifestyle advice, or point her in the direction of someone who can (see Resources). With her family history, DEXA is a good idea. Given her age, systemic HRT at this point would not be wise, but vaginal HRT is likely to help her presenting symptoms. The long-term use of low-dose vaginal oestrogens on the endometrium is uncertain, but you will be seeing her again after her scan.

What do you prescribe?

Topical (vaginal) oestrogens come in the form of **tablets** (Vagifem), pessaries (Ortho-Gynest), intravaginal **creams** (Gynest and Ovestin) and a **vaginal ring** (Estring).

General Practice Cases at a Glance, First Edition. Carol Cooper and Martin L Block. © 2017 John Wiley & Sons, Ltd. Published 2017 by John Wiley & Sons, Ltd.

You end up prescribing Vagifem once nightly for the first week, then twice weekly at night. You tell her she won't absorb much of the hormone into the bloodstream. She then asks, 'Can he absorb any of it?'

How do you reply?

Yes, this can happen, so it is best to avoid using the tablet before sex. Explain that intercourse reduces the woman's absorption of the hormone, and exposes the man to the risk of absorbing it instead. Over time, this could be harmful.

One way of avoiding this risk would be to schedule the use of the tablet. Another would be to use condoms. There is no evidence that Vagifem damages latex.

What other important topic should you cover today?

You should discuss safe sex. STIs are rising in the over-50s, one reason being that this age group no longer uses contraception. You can tell Mrs Fraser that many common sexually transmitted infections cause no symptoms, so there's no way of telling who has or hasn't got one. Many infections like chlamydia can be carried for a long time, only to cause trouble later. She and her new man should consider a check at the sexual health clinic.

She replies that she wouldn't want to do that, for fear of embarrassment. You tell her there is no shame attached to the clinic, and that people of all ages and walks of life attend. She is still unconvinced, so you decide to shelve the topic until you see her again.

Resources

FRAX: WHO Fracture Risk Assessment Tool.
  https://www.shef.ac.uk/FRAX/
National Osteoporosis Society (charity with information for the public and professionals).
  www.nos.org.uk
British National Formulary.
Hurst BS, Jones AI, Elliot M, *et al*. Absorption of vaginal estrogen cream during sexual intercourse: a prospective, randomized, controlled trial. *J Reprod Med*. 2008; 53(1): 29–32.
  http://www.ncbi.nlm.nih.gov/pubmed/18251358

CASE

24 I've got a bit of a discharge

Suzy Fox, age 19 years
Student
PMH: IBS
Medication: Microgynon; cetirizine every
spring/summer

While attending for her Pill check, Suzy says she has a vaginal discharge. She's not sure exactly when it began, but she went to Ibiza a month ago with two of her friends and had sex with 'a couple of people' without using condoms. She has a boyfriend who did not go on this holiday. He has no symptoms but she wonders if she 'caught something'. Her discharge is thick and white, and very itchy. There's no smell and it sounds like thrush to you.

Based on what you've heard so far, can you reassure her?

No. Her symptoms are likely to be due to thrush, which is not a sexually transmitted infection (STI), contrary to popular opinion. However she is at risk of an STI, and her partner is therefore also at risk.

Causes of vaginal discharge

Common infections
- Bacterial vaginosis (affects 30% of women with discharge).
- *Candida* (another 30%).
Note that neither of these is sexually transmitted, but they are much more common in the sexually active.

STIs
- *Chlamydia* (very common).
- Gonorrhoea (less common).
- *Trichomonas vaginalis* (less common).

Non-infective
- Physiological (common).
- Cervical ectopy or polyps.
- Retained tampon.
- Malignancy (e.g. vulval, cervical).
- Allergies.
- Vesicovaginal or rectovaginal fistula.

Which STIs can be asymptomatic? Write down at least six.

- *Chlamydia* – 10% of women aged 16–19 have it. Asymptomatic in 70% of women and over 50% of men (possibly even 90%).
- *Trichomonas vaginalis* (TV) – asymptomatic in up to 50% of men and women.
- Gonorrhoea – asymptomatic in up to 50% of women (depending on site of infection) and 20% of men.
- Syphilis.
- Genital herpes simplex.
- HPV – asymptomatic in up to 90%.

- HIV.
- Hepatitis B.
This is almost all of them.

You tell Suzy that she could possibly have caught an STI.

Tip

Be as non-judgemental as you can. Every doctor brings their own beliefs and standards to any consultation, but being genuinely patient-centred means putting these to one side. Avoid indicating that she may have been stupid. Also avoid suggesting that you might have done the same as her.

You decide to prescribe for her presumed Candida infection. What do you prescribe and in what dose?

Both vaginal and oral azoles work well, so it depends on patient preference (but avoid oral treatment in pregnancy). Clotrimazole pessary 500 mg (single dose) inserted at night is a good choice, combined with clotrimazole cream to relieve vulval itching. Note that these vaginal treatments can damage latex. Alternatives are fluconazole 150 mg (single dose) orally or itraconazole 400 mg as two doses 12 hours apart.

Remember to check her BP and prescribe the Pill she came in for.

You are concerned about the possibility of an STI. What do you do now?

(a) Test in the practice?
(b) Advise her to go to the GUM clinic?
Either is acceptable, and the GUM clinic does not have to be her nearest one. Many practices can test for the range of STIs, while others may struggle. Or the patient may have a preference. One important issue is timely, accurate and sensitive diagnosis. Another is partner notification (i.e. contact tracing).

Tip

Note that GUM clinics offer free treatment, while patients may need to pay a prescription charge in primary care.

Testing for STIs

As a minimum, if you offer testing you should test for *Chlamydia*, gonorrhoea, *Trichomonas*, and syphilis (RCGP Guidelines 2006).
- *Chlamydia* and gonorrhoea: nucleic acid amplification tests (NAATs) are the best screening test, on either urine, self-taken vaginal swab or endocervical swab.
- *Trichomonas*: HVS.
- Syphilis: serology.
Note: managing gonorrhoea or syphilis is complex, so, if diagnosed, refer promptly to GUM for treatment.

Does she need an HIV test?

Yes, she probably does, and you can test as it is four weeks after contact. Heterosexual spread is not common but it is rising. The sooner HIV is diagnosed, the better the outcome. General practices can easily do this, and specialist counselling is unnecessary. The more normalized HIV testing becomes, the more infections will be picked up at an early stage.

Tip

Terrence Higgins Trust and various other organizations offer walk-in HIV testing services. See www.tht.org.uk.

You may want to discuss and explore her hepatitis B risk since she had unprotected sex with a couple of partners in a place where hep B is common and IV drug use is prevalent. She may have already been vaccinated, in which case you may wish to consider checking her immune status, as she may need a booster.

You discuss all this with Suzy. She thinks on balance she will go to the GUM clinic, as she has heard you can be anonymous.

What one piece of advice must you give her?

She must **use condoms** or **abstain from sex** until she knows from the tests that she isn't putting her partner at risk. Many women with thrush find sex too painful, but not all. Remember that vaginal treatments for thrush can damage latex.

If Suzy has not told her boyfriend about her other sexual contacts, she may find it hard to explain to him why she suddenly wants to use a barrier method. It is unwise to collude with a patient and help concoct a lie. But you could suggest she studies the Pill leaflet carefully and makes up her own mind as to what might be convincing in her situation.

In terms of her future health, she would benefit from advice on safer sex.

Resources

Sexually transmitted infections in primary care 2013 RCGP and
    BASHH.
    http://www.bashh.org/documents/Sexually%20Transmitted%
    20Infections%20in%20Primary%20Care%202013.pdf
CKS: HIV infection and AIDS.
    http://cks.nice.org.uk/hiv-infection-and-aids#!diagnosissub:8
HIV in Primary Care (2011).
    www.medfash.org.uk
For patients: NHS Choices.
    http://www.nhs.uk/Livewell/Talkingaboutsex/Pages/
    Ineedhelpnow.aspx

CASE

25 I'm feeling tired and woozy

Home visit

Gladys O'Sullivan, age 84 years

Retired. Carer for her husband John O'Sullivan, 85, who has significant RA

PMH: hypertension; hypothyroidism

Medication: amlodipine 5 mg daily, levothyroxine 75 µg daily

Gladys O'Sullivan is on today's visit request book. The surgery took a call from her husband. The message says Mrs O'Sullivan is tired and confused. You return the call and speak to Mr O'Sullivan who tells you that he is worried about his wife. He tells you his wife has been increasingly tired over the last couple of days. Today she seems a little confused and forgetful (which is not really like her). He would be very grateful for a visit. You tell Mr O'Sullivan you will visit them after morning surgery.

Mrs O'Sullivan greets you at the door. She is still wearing her dressing gown and no make-up. This is most unlike her. She does, however, recognize you as her doctor.

What are the important areas you need to explore here in your history?

In this case it is key to:
- define the **problem**
- define the **impact** it is having on both of them both.

What questions would you ask to define the problem?

Begin with some open questions, which give Mr and Mrs O'Sullivan a chance to describe fully what has been going on. Often something simple like, 'Tell me what has been going on?' works well. You may need to clarify further with some closed questions if you need more detail here.

There are some specifics that it would be useful to enquire about.
- Any other symptoms (such as pain, shortness of breath, urinary symptoms)?
- Any fever?
- Has there been any fall or head injury?
- What is her normal sate of functioning?
It would be useful to get a sense of the **level of confusion**. This can be done directly assessing Mrs O'Sullivan by assessing her orientation in time, place and person.
- **Time:** What day is it? What season are we in?
- **Place:** Where are we? What town?
- **Person:** Who am I?
Just as important will be Mr O'Sullivan's description of the pattern and fluctuation here.

Mrs O'Sullivan says that she feels really tired and 'woozy'. Mr O'Sullivan says that she did seem to have a temperature last night and that she was getting up to go to the toilet several times in the night. This is unlike her. There has been no fall or head injury. Mrs

O'Sullivan seems slower cognitively that usual. She's not sure what day it is or what month, but she knows she is at home and that you are her doctor.

How are you going to define the impact of this problem? Write down some questions to ask.

Again, begin with something simple. 'How is this illness affecting you?' is a nice clear open question that should give you plenty of useful information. However it will be useful to be clear about some specifics here.
- 'Have you been able to look after yourself?'
- 'How about eating?'
- 'What about washing and dressing?'
- 'Do you normally get any help at home?'
- 'Any friends or family who have been helping out the last couple of days?'
This is doubly important as Mrs O'Sullivan cares for her husband. He has significant RA with severe deformity affecting his hands, is unable to cook or prepare food, and needs a little help with washing and dressing. They do not usually have any help at home.

Mrs O'Sullivan is quite hesitant when talking about these things today. Mr O'Sullivan is helpful in explaining more. He tells you that neither of them have got changed out of their night clothes for the last couple of days. Yesterday they had some bread and jam for lunch. They have only eaten a few biscuits since then.

Mrs O'Sullivan starts to cry at this point, and looks ashamed.

What is your differential diagnosis?

Acute confusion – differential diagnosis

Acute infections
- Urinary tract infection.
- Pneumonia.
- Viral infections.
- Meningitis.

Prescribed drugs
- Benzodiazepines.
- Analgesics, e.g. morphine.

Toxic substances
- E.g. alcohol – acute intoxication or withdrawal.

Vascular disorders
- Cerebrovascular haemorrhage or infarction.
- Cardiac failure or ischaemia.
- Subdural haemorrhage.
- Subarachnoid haemorrhage.

Metabolic causes
- Hypoxia.
- Electrolyte abnormalities, e.g. hyponatraemia and hypercalcaemia.
- Hypoglycaemia or hyperglycaemia.

General Practice Cases at a Glance, First Edition. Carol Cooper and Martin L Block. © 2017 John Wiley & Sons, Ltd. Published 2017 by John Wiley & Sons, Ltd.

- Hepatic impairment.
- Renal impairment.

Endocrinopathies
- Hypothyroidism.
- Hyperthyroidism.

Trauma
- Head injury.

Neoplasia
- Primary cerebral malignancy.

Others
- Urinary retention.
- Faecal impaction.

What examination would you like to do? Name these specifically before continuing.

In this case a full physical examination would be useful to add to your assessment of her mental state.

Your findings are as follows:
- Temperature 37.7 °C.
- Pulse 88 regular.
- BP 134/69.
- Oxygen sats 98% on air.
- Blood glucose 4.8 mmol/L.
- CVS: heart sounds normal, pulse regular.
- Respiratory rate 14/minute; chest clear.
- Abdomen soft and non-tender.
- Neuro – cranial nerves intact; peripheral nervous system normal tone, power and reflexes; gait a little slow but steady.
- Urine dipstick: leucocytes ++, nitrites +.

What is the likely diagnosis here?

Her history of increase in urinary frequency, mild confusion and tiredness, combined with her mild temperature and urine findings all point to a diagnosis of UTI.

What are you going to do?

You need to think how you will treat this condition. You need to send an **MSU** and prescribe **antibiotics** (e.g. trimethoprim 200 mg bd for seven days), but you also need to consider her and her husband's **safety and welfare.**

Mrs O'Sullivan doesn't want to go to hospital. Mr O'Sullivan is very worried about how they are going to cope right now.

Any thoughts as to what to do next?

This may be a case where you can contact your local **Rapid Response team** (or equivalent). They can arrange for an urgent care package to be put in place to help with meals and self-care and regular nurse review to check in on progress.

You call your local Rapid Response team. The lead nurse comes out within the next 2 hours, along with a carer. The O'Sullivans get a hot meal and a short-term package of care is put in place for both of them.

You pop in a couple of days later to find that Mrs O'Sullivan is looking and feeling much improved. She is grateful for your help and really happy that you managed to keep her out of hospital.

Resources
CKS/NICE Delerium.
   http://cks.nice.org.uk/delirium

I think I need to get my blood pressure checked

Susan Braithwaite, age 53 years

School teacher

PMH: nil

Medication: nil

Susan Braithwaite comes to see you. She is not someone who comes to the doctor very often. Today she tells you that she has just been to sign up at the gym, and they have told her to see the nurse because her blood pressure is high. She saw the nurse, who recorded her BP readings as 166/88, 169/84 and 155/104. The nurse arranged blood tests and asked her to book in to see the GP. Mrs Braithwaite is very surprised by all this, as she feels completely well.

The bloods performed by the nurse show normal renal function, an Hba1c of 34 mmol/mol (5.3%), a total cholesterol of 5.6 mmol/L with an HDL:LDL ratio of 3.0.

You check Mrs Braithwaite's blood pressure three times. The readings are 172/104, 164/95 and 164/93.

What lifestyle factors are worth enquiring about? Write down at least four.

- Smoking.
- Diet.
- Exercise.
- Alcohol intake.
- Stress levels.

Smoking, poor diet, lack of exercise, high alcohol intake and stress can all contribute to an increase in blood pressure.

Mrs Braithwaite is Afro-Caribbean. She tells you that she has smoked 20 cigarettes a day since she was a teenager. She has tried stopping a couple of times over the years but with no success. She does her best to eat healthily, eating lots of fruit and vegetables. She walks regularly, but this is quite gentle exercise and she was hoping to improve on this by joining the gym. She drinks 7–10 units of alcohol a week. Her work can get pretty stressful, she says, though right now things are OK.

What other area should you cover in your history?

Family history is important. Does she have a family history of hypertension, ischaemic heart disease, stroke or diabetes?

She tells you that her father died of a heart attack in his 70s. He had high blood pressure. Her older brother has type 2 diabetes and high blood pressure.

Can you confirm the diagnosis of hypertension right now?

NICE guidance advises that, if the patient's BP is 140/90 or greater on **two or three** occasions in clinic, you should confirm this with either:

- home BP reading; or
- ambulatory readings (24-hour BP).

You arrange for Mrs Braithwaite to have the practice's 24 hour BP device fitted and review her with the results.

Table 26.1 Stage 1 and stage 2 hypertension.

Stage 1 hypertension
Clinic blood pressure is above or equal to 140/90 mmHg, and ABPM average is above or equal to 135/85 mmHg
Treat based on an assessment of the total cardiovascular disease risk, treating 10-year CVD risk scores greater than 20%

Stage 2 hypertension
Clinic blood pressure is above or equal to 160/100 mmHg, and ABPM average is above or equal to 150/95 mmHg, or there is isolated systolic hypertension with a systolic blood pressure of 160 mmHg or higher
Treat with antihypertensive medication

Mrs Braithwaite returns to see you, and her ambulatory BP readings are consistent with her clinic readings. Her average daytime blood pressure is 164/92.

What is the diagnosis?

Mrs Braithwaite has a new diagnosis of hypertension. She has stage 2 hypertension (Table 26.1).

For Mrs Braithwaite's long-term wellbeing, it is vital that she understands her diagnosis and its implications. Here the clarity of your explanation is really important.

As well as confirming the diagnosis with ambulatory or home BP readings, what other tests should you be arranging now?

Patient **weight** – in this case 68 kg, giving her a BMI of 26.

Arrange further baseline investigations to complete your **risk factor assessments** and to assess **end-organ damage**.

- Risk factor assessment: lipid profile and Hba1c for diabetes (this has already been done in this case by the nurse).
- End-organ damage assessment:
  - ECG
  - U+Es
  - **urine** dipstick for protein – if positive send off for testing for albumin:creatinine ratio; this is an important sign of renal damage, and if raised it would lower your target BP for treatment
  - **fundoscopy.**

How would you explain a new diagnosis of hypertension to Mrs Braithwaite?

Find an explanation that feels natural to you and is clear and avoids medical jargon. An example might be, 'Your blood pressure is a measure of the pressure in your blood vessels. We know that if this becomes higher it can cause damage to the blood vessels and increase your chances of getting disease of some of your vital organs, like the heart, the brain and the kidneys.'

It's good to check with the patient at this point to see if she has any questions. You should then go on to explain the reason for lowering the blood pressure, for example, 'We know that if you bring high blood pressure down, it lowers the chances of damage to the heart, brain and kidneys.' It's worth practising a couple of explanations here, to find your natural style.

General Practice Cases at a Glance, First Edition. Carol Cooper and Martin L Block. © 2017 John Wiley & Sons, Ltd. Published 2017 by John Wiley & Sons, Ltd.

Don't underestimate the importance of your explanation at this stage. Hypertension is a chronic condition, and if Mrs Braithwaite leaves without a good understanding of it, she is less likely to follow through with any treatment. Often a patient information leaflet is helpful here, or you could refer her to a website like the British Heart Foundation's.

What should your management be?

- Lifestyle advice.
- Antihypertensive medication.
- Consider a statin.

Lifestyle

The most single most important thing here is stopping **smoking**, and it is really worth emphasizing this. Smoking is a major risk factor for cardiovascular disease. Adding smoking to hypertension exponentially increases her cardiovascular risk. She would benefit from increasing her exercise level (e.g. brisk exercise for 30–60 minutes, three to five times a week). She would be safe to join the gym but you should encourage her to build up her exercise level gradually initially. The practice nurse will be able to offer her smoking cessation help, and this will increase her chance of successfully quitting. Her **BMI** of 26 is also a little high. You should discuss this as bringing it down, through diet and exercise, is likely to improve her BP.

Antihypertensive medication

As she has stage 2 hypertension, she would benefit from treatment with antihypertensive medication. You should refer to NICE guidance in choosing your agent.

The guidance recommends that people who are 55 years of age or older, and those who are of black African or Caribbean ethnic origin (of any age), should be offered a calcium-channel blocker, e.g. amlodipine 5 mg. Mrs Braithwaite's ethnicity is Afro-Caribbean. **The target BP is 140/90.**

Choice of antihypertensive medication

- People who are **younger than 55 years of age** and not of black African or Caribbean ethnic origin, start an angiotensin-converting enzyme inhibitor (**ACE inhibitor**).
- People who are **55 years of age or older** and those who are of **black African or Caribbean ethnic origin** (of any age) should be offered a **calcium-channel blocker**.
- If not tolerated or if has heart failure, offer a thiazide diuretic, e.g. bendroflumethiazide 2.5 mg daily.

Consider a statin

If her 10-year CVD risk is >20% she would benefit from a statin (e.g. atorvastatin 20 mg daily). Calculate her CVD risk using a tool such as QRisk (qrisk.org). These use parameters such as the patient's age, gender, BMI, smoking status, diabetic status and cholesterol ratio to calculate a 10-year risk of developing cardiovascular disease. It is worth checking you have up-to-date values of all these readings before treating. Using the readings from the recent bloods taken by the nurse the QRisk calculator gives your patient a 10-year CVD risk of 6.7%. She therefore does not need a statin.

At the end of the consultation, Mrs Braithwaite agrees to see the nurse to talk about her smoking and leaves with a prescription for amlodipine 5 mg. She will be returning to see you in a month for a repeat BP.

Resources

NICE (2011a) Hypertension. Clinical management of primary hypertension in adults (NICE guideline). Clinical guidance 127. National Institute for Health and Care Excellence. www.nice.org.uk

online CV risk calculator. www.qrisk.org

CASE

27

Well, I'm pregnant

Elena Marcovich, age 24 years

Nanny/childminder

PMH: TOP 8 months ago; chondromalacia patellae in her teens

Medication: nil

Elena Marcovich did a pregnancy test yesterday. The test was positive, and she says she wants 'to get rid of it'. She is a live-in nanny, with no place of her own, and she says there is no way she can have a child right now.

She was on the Pill in the past, but often forgot to take it, hence her unplanned pregnancy last year. She and her boyfriend had been using condoms, and she fell pregnant despite this.

What do you want to find out from her now? Write down at least two questions.

- Ask for her **LMP** and details of her **usual cycle**, to establish how pregnant she is.
- Find out about her **last TOP**: when, how and were there any after-effects. It is surprising that she did not start an effective method of contraception then. Perhaps this was not discussed properly, or perhaps she failed to take it seriously. Some gentle questioning here may help clarify.
- Explore **why** she wants a termination. She may be in an unstable relationship. ► Is there any element of pressure here? She may have conceived as a result of rape, or of sex with her employer. A request for a TOP should not be met with resistance, but it is an opportunity to find out if there has been any coercion or violence. An open non-judgemental question like, 'Can you tell me a bit more about why you want an abortion?' may unlock doors. Importantly, you must also establish whether a termination would be in line with the Abortion Act.
- Ask '**What does your boyfriend think?**' Of course a woman can have a termination without her partner's approval. However his knowledge and involvement can support her in her decision. She has to make her own choices, but your job as a GP is to help her explore all the options and make the choice she is least likely to regret later.

From her LMP she is five weeks pregnant. Her cycle is regular, 5/29, and periods are heavy. Her last TOP was a suction TOP (STOP) on the NHS. Afterwards she took the Pill again for a short time, then gave up. She has a regular boyfriend 'more or less'. He is supportive of her having an abortion, and she herself has 'no doubts at all' about termination. Of course she likes children, she says, but it is wrong for her to have a child now and she says she could not handle it. She also suspects she would lose her job. Her employer is a single mother.

Summary of the Abortion Act 1967

Termination before 24 weeks of gestation is allowed if it:
- reduces the risk to a woman's life; or
- reduces the risk to her physical or mental health; or

- reduces the risk to physical or mental health of her existing children; or
- if the baby is at substantial risk of being seriously mentally or physically handicapped.

Because of improvements in neonatal medicine, there is debate about whether to reduce the upper limit from 24 weeks of gestation to 22 or even 20. Note that there is no upper limit if termination is done to save the woman's life, or for risk of grave permanent injury to the mother's physical/mental health, or if there is 'substantial risk' that, if the child were born, it would suffer such physical or mental abnormalities as to be seriously handicapped.

► If the conditions are not met, then abortion remains a criminal offence under the Offences Against the Persons Act 1861.

She asks if she can have 'the abortion pill'.

Is she suitable for medical termination?

Yes. Medical abortion is now considered appropriate at almost any gestation.

Medical termination of pregnancy

Over half of all TOPs in England are now medical rather than suction terminations.

Medical abortion: mifepristone plus prostaglandin, e.g. mifepristone 200 mg orally followed 36–48 hours later by misoprostol 800 μg by vaginal, buccal or sublingual route. Repeat doses of misoprostol (often 400 μg but dose varies with gestation) may be needed after 4 hours.

The regime is safe, effective (6 in 1000 failure rate as compared to 2 in 1000 for surgical TOP), and considered to have no adverse impact on future pregnancies.

It is wise to give a woman breathing space, and, at five weeks' gestation, time is on her side. You ask if she would like to think it over until tomorrow or the day after, and come back to see you. But she says no, she has made up her mind. You therefore agree to refer her for termination.

What three tests should she have before any kind of termination?

- The **pregnancy** should be confirmed, and shown to be **uterine**, so a scan is needed.
- You need to find out if she is **rhesus negative**.
- She should have a **chlamydia test**.

You do not need to do these tests yourself. In your referral note, give whatever information you have, and mention which tests you have or have not done.

What two further areas must you cover before she leaves your consulting room?

- Discuss her choices re future **contraception.**
- A warning that she may feel **sad or regretful** after the termination.

Table 27.1 Long-acting reversible contraception methods.

Method	Failure rate	How long it lasts	Use after TOP	Notes
Implant of etonorgestrel (single rod)	<0.1% at 3 years	3 years	Can be used immediately after TOP	Irregular bleeding common
Levonorgestrel-releasing IUS	0.1% at 1 year	5 years (Mirena) 3 years (Jaydess, which is a lower dose)	Can be used immediately after first-trimester TOP	May take 7 days to take effect Reduces menstrual blood loss; often causes amenorrhoea
Depot injection of medroxyprogesterone acetate or norethisterone enanthate	0.3% at 1 year	12 weeks (medroxyprogesterone); 8 weeks (norethisterone)	Can be used immediately after TOP	Takes 7 days to take effect Irregular bleeding common
Copper IUCD	0.6% at 1 year	5–10 years	Can be used immediately after first-trimester TOP	Heavy bleeding +/– dysmenorrhoea can occur

Elena is likely to be at the peak of her fertility and has yet to find the right method of contraception for herself. She may want to continue with condoms to protect against STI, but even with the most meticulous use their failure rate is at least 2 per 100 woman years.

She admits she is not good at taking the Pill, so long-acting reversible contraception (LARC) might be more suitable. In view of her heavy periods, she might prefer the IUS, and may want to avoid the implant and depot injections, but the final choice is hers.

Make sure you document her choice, if any, on your referral note. Even if the clinic deals with her contraception, she should see you for follow-up post-TOP.

LARC

All LARCs are cost effective, with a failure rate less than one in 100 at one year. According to some data, they are less expensive at one year than the oral contraceptive Pill. Obesity does not contraindicate LARC unless there is established cardiovascular disease or other serious problems.

Although you may not offer all the options in Table 27.1 yourself, you should know about them to be able to inform your patient and offer the full choice.

Resources

GMC: Personal beliefs and medical practice (2013).
http://www.gmc-uk.org/guidance/ethical_guidance/21171.asp
NICE guideline: Long-acting reversible contraception CG30.
http://www.nice.org.uk/Guidance/CG30
FPA: your guide to contraception.
http://www.fpa.org.uk/contraception-help/your-guide-contraception
You may also like to try Case 39: 'I don't want to have my period when I am on holiday'.

CASE
28 I've been feeling short of breath

> **Mary McArthur, age 63 years**
>
> Retired
>
> Ex-smoker (20/day) – gave up three years ago
>
> PMH: moderate COPD
>
> Medication: salbutamol inhaler 100 μg 2 puffs qds prn, Salmeterol inhaler 50 μg 1 puff bd
>
> Most recent spirometry: FEV1 62% predicted; FEV1/FVC ratio 64%

Mrs McArthur is seeing you during your morning emergency clinic. You call her in from your waiting room and she follows you to your room. She doesn't look herself and by the time she sits down in your consulting room you can hear she is wheezing. You give her a moment to catch her breath and then ask her what you can do for her today.

Mrs McArthur goes on to tell you that over the past few days she has been feeling more unwell. It started with a cough and a cold, but over the past two days she has been feeling increasingly short of breath on exertion. She is normally able to walk around the house and up to the shops and back without any problems, but today and yesterday she is finding that if she walks a short distance she starts feeling wheezy and has to take a rest. She even felt a little breathless walking up your corridor. She is bringing up some thick green phlegm too.

What is the most likely diagnosis here?

It is likely that Mrs McArthur has an acute infective exacerbation of COPD.

What other questions should you ask to be clear about the diagnosis?

Find out about any **chest pain**, to rule out other possible cardiac or respiratory causes of her breathlessness. In cardiac ischaemia you would expect a heavy central chest pain on exertion, or at rest, and in pulmonary embolism you might expect a pleuritic chest pain on inspiration. You should also ask about the presence of **fever**. If this is persisting, it would point towards a bacterial infection. Clarify what her normal **sputum** production is like. A change in the level of purulence of sputum may be an indicator of bacterial infection.

Mrs McArthur has no other symptoms. There is no pain, and though there was a little fever at the beginning this has settled now.

What other questions should you ask to be clear about her safety?

Get a sense of how she is coping and the impact this exacerbation is having on her. If she is not able to cope or if she is alone then she may be a candidate for a hospital admission (see box: When to consider hospital admission).

Mrs McArthur tells you that she is coping OK. Michael has been doing the shopping and keeping an eye on her. Her daughter Jane lives round the corner with her family and pops over every night after work to check in on her.

What examination should you perform and what simple practice test should you do?

Mrs McArthur should have a respiratory and cardiovascular examination. This should also include her vital signs. You should also take an oxygen saturation level.

- Pulse 88 regular.
- Temperature 36.7 °C.
- BP 138/83.
- Oxygen saturation level is 94% on air.

Her chest has wheeze throughout. There are no crackles and no signs of an effusion. Heart sounds are normal. No oedema.

What is the diagnosis?

Mrs McArthur does indeed have an acute infective exacerbation of COPD.

Should she be treated at home or should she be admitted to hospital?

Even though she is troubled by her symptoms, there are no features in her history or on examination to suggest this is a severe exacerbation that needs admission (see box). She can be treated at home. Besides, Mrs McArthur is very keen not to go to hospital. She hates hospitals.

> **When to consider hospital admission**
>
> Consider hospital admission if any of the following are present.
> - Severe breathlessness, rapid onset, confusion, cyanosis, worsening peripheral oedema or impaired consciousness.
> - The person is unable to cope or lives alone.
> - Their general condition is poor or deteriorating (poor activity, confined to bed, or on long-term oxygen therapy).
> - Significant comorbidity (particularly cardiac disease or type 1 diabetes mellitus).
> - A low oxygen saturation (less than 90%).
>
> From CKS NICE COPD.

What should your management be?

- Maximize **inhaler** treatment. Mrs McArthur should be encouraged to use her salbutamol inhaler regularly over the next few days, two puffs four times daily.
- Give **steroids**. As she has shortness of breath that interferes with daily activities, she should be prescribed prednisolone 30 mg od for 7–14 days.
- Prescribe **antibiotics**. If there is a history of increasingly purulent sputum or signs of bacterial pneumonia she should be given amoxicillin 500 mg three times daily (refer to your local guidance).

What about other health promotion or management of this continuing problem? Is there anything else you would like to cover?

She should have an annual flu vaccination and a one-off pneumonia vaccination.

You should consider offering pulmonary rehabilitation too. This is an exercise-based programme that is useful in COPD patients. It is offered to patients who have ongoing functional impairment due to their COPD. Mrs McArthur may be about to reach this point.

Tip

As a general principle, it is a good idea in GP consultations to think not just about the acute presentation but also:
- managing the **chronic disease** (in this case on-going COPD care)
- **health promotion** where appropriate.

What safety net should you put in place?

There are two aspects that one needs to consider here:
- safety netting against a deterioration in condition that requires further medical input
- safety netting against persisting symptoms which suggest another diagnosis.

In relation to the first point, you should advise her to contact a doctor if she is suffering from increasing shortness of breath, if she is struggling to manage at home or becoming increasingly unwell.

It is also important to talk about persisting symptoms. If she is still feeling short of breath at the end of treatment she should be reassessed. Likewise if she is still coughing in three weeks time she would need a chest x-ray to rule out malignancy.

Diagnosis of COPD

It is important to consider the diagnosis of COPD in patients who have features suggesting this as outlined in the box.

COPD diagnosis

COPD diagnosis can be made if:
- age older than 35 years
- has a risk factor (smoker, ex-smoker, or occupational exposure)
- typical symptoms: exertional breathlessness, chronic cough, regular sputum production, frequent 'winter bronchitis', wheeze
- absence of clinical features of asthma
- presence of airflow obstruction confirmed by post-bronchodilator spirometry
- FEV1/FVC ratio is less than 0.7.

The diagnosis is confirmed by spirometry, which is done by the practice nurse. Although the FEV1/FVC is useful in confirming diagnosis, it is the FEV1 predicted percentage which gives us a guide as to disease severity and progression. Mrs McArthur has moderate COPD as shown by her FEV1 of 62% predicted.

Classification of severity of COPD in relation to FEV1 at spirometry

Stage 1 – mild: FEV1 80% of predicted value or higher (symptoms must be present).

Stage 2 – moderate: FEV1 50–79% of predicted value.

Stage 3 – severe: FEV1 30–49% of predicted value.

Stage 4 – very severe: FEV1 less than 30% of predicted value.

Resources

CKS/NICE Chronic Obstructive Pulmonary Disease.
http://cks.nice.org.uk/chronic-obstructive-pulmonary-disease

CASE
29
She's coughing non-stop

Josie West, age 3 years
PMH: croup
Medication: nil

Josie has had a cough for three weeks, as her mother explains. It's worse at night, and it's making her so tired, it's 'wearing her out'. Otherwise Josie is fairly well, not off her food and hasn't had a cold recently. Mrs West tried some cough syrup but it didn't help.

Josie is an only child and attends a Montessori school. Her immunizations are up to date. There's no family history of asthma.

What are your initial thoughts? Write down at least four possibilities.

- **URTI** is the most common cause of cough in a child, but Josie is well and has no other symptoms.
- **Asthma** affects around 15% of children, and can be severe, even fatal. Wheeze is often absent.
- **Inhaled foreign body** would probably have caused secondary infection by now.
- **Pneumonia** is very not likely as Josie appears well.
- **Pertussis** can still occur in 5% of children despite immunization. Cough usually occurs in paroxysms.
- **Epiglottitis** is now rare in children, thanks to Hib vaccine.

From the history so far, either URTI or asthma are most likely, but always think about FB and ask about ▶ choking and ▶ whether symptoms began abruptly.

You examine Josie. She is coughing a little. Her temperature is normal and RR is 25. There is no stridor, and no intercostal or subcostal recession but with your stethoscope you can hear mild wheezing bilaterally. Her throat and TMs are normal. She looks about the right size for her age, and measurements confirm she is around the 50th percentile for height, and just below it for weight. Pulse oximetry is 98%.

Key point
Whenever you see a child, always ask yourself 'Is this child ill?'

What further useful questions could you ask? Write down three.

- 'Does Josie often **wheeze**?' If necessary, explain what this sounds like.
- 'Does she cough or wheeze when she does **exercise** like running, or when she's **laughing**?'
- 'Is she allergic to anything?' Also ask about hay fever and other allergies in the family.
- 'Does anyone in your home **smoke**?' Even smoking in a different room can affect a child as smoke clings to clothes and soft furnishings. Ask too about anyone who looks after Josie.
- 'Are there **pets** at home?' Animals are a common trigger of allergic asthma.
- 'Has **anything changed** recently?' Allergens can persist for up to 18 months or more, so a house move can be relevant. Or you may uncover a source of stress.

Mrs West has occasionally heard Josie wheeze when she's running around in the park. Nobody smokes. Mrs West has hay fever badly but is not aware of other allergies in the immediate family. There are no pets, and they have lived at the same address since before Josie was born.

What is your working diagnosis and what do you tell the mother?

It's probably asthma, but it could be URTI. You tell the mother it's likely to be asthma, although it might turn out to be just a virus.

Key point
UK has one of the highest rates of childhood asthma in the world. About 1.1 m children in UK currently get treatment for asthma.

The National Review of Asthma Deaths (2014) found that the overall standard of care for young children and young people was inadequate. In almost half of asthma deaths in children, it was well below expected standards. **Every doctor who deals with children who have asthma needs to maintain clinical standards.**

What do you do now?

Your choice is either to do nothing and review her in a few days, or to prescribe a trial of bronchodilator. You decide to prescribe.

Write down what you would now prescribe.

Salbutamol MDI (metered dose inhaler, Figure 29.1) is suitable, for use up to four times daily. Include a spacer device, e.g. Aerochamber, which is medium-sized, or Volumatic, which is larger. At three years, Josie would probably cope with a mouthpiece, but you could prescribe a mask and see which she manages best.

How will Josie learn to use the inhaler?

Even in families with asthma, don't assume parents know the right way to operate inhalers. Ideally you or your practice nurse would teach Josie how to use the inhaler and spacer. But the pharmacist is also well placed to do this, in which case you can bring Josie and her mother back in a day or two for the nurse to check the technique.

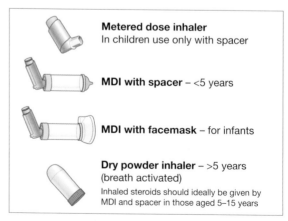

Metered dose inhaler
In children use only with spacer

MDI with spacer – <5 years

MDI with facemask – for infants

Dry powder inhaler – >5 years
(breath activated)
Inhaled steroids should ideally be given by MDI and spacer in those aged 5–15 years

Figure 29.1 Some inhaler devices.

General Practice Cases at a Glance, First Edition. Carol Cooper and Martin L Block. © 2017 John Wiley & Sons, Ltd. Published 2017 by John Wiley & Sons, Ltd.

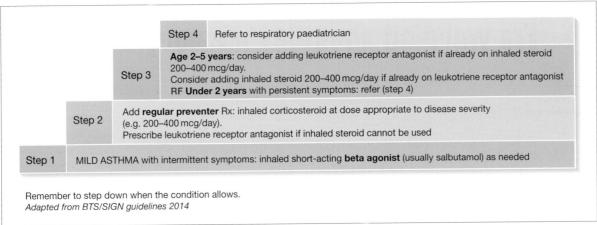

Figure 29.2 Stepwise management of asthma in children under five years. Adapted from BTS/SIGN guidelines, 2014.

Josie returns in 10 days to see you. She is using the inhaler about twice a day. Her mother says she's no longer coughing. She's also more alert at her little school, and can run about without wheezing or getting out of breath.

What do you do next?

You can tell the mother that this clinches the diagnosis of asthma. It is likely to be mild, but all the same the family needs to know all about asthma. Consider a **management plan card**, such as the one from charity Asthma UK, in which to write down what Josie should take. The card also lists the symptoms of worsening asthma.

Consider the need for adding a regular dose of 'preventer' medication, in the form of inhaled corticosteroid 200-400 μg/day in two daily doses. This would be the next step in the management according to the British Thoracic Society/SIGN guidelines (Figures 29.2, 29.3). However you have only just made Josie's diagnosis, so you can allow some time on a PRN dose of 'reliever' and review her in 2–3 months.

Josie and her mother return in exactly two months. Josie has needed an inhaler every day, sometimes twice daily. You mention a regular dose of steroid as a 'preventer' but Mrs West is not keen.

What can you say to address her concerns?

Find out exactly what she is worried about. Some people confuse steroid inhalers with anabolic steroids. Parents may also be concerned about infections, weight gain or poor growth. You can reassure Mrs West that untreated or under-treated asthma is more likely to cause poor growth than steroids do. There are however ways of reducing unwanted effects from steroids: using a spacer, and brushing the teeth or rinsing the mouth immediately after the inhaler. Explain that you will follow Josie up, and there is always the possibility of reducing medication in future, depending on how she is. Again, Asthma UK can help inform and reassure parents and carers.

Resources

CKS/NICE Asthma.
   http://cks.nice.org.uk/asthma#!topicsummary
BTS/SIGN guidelines on asthma (last update 2014).
   www.brit-thoracic.org.uk/document-library/clinical-information/
   asthma/btssign-asthma-guideline-quick-reference-guide-2014/
Asthma UK: information on asthma for families; asthma action plan.
   www.asthma.org.uk

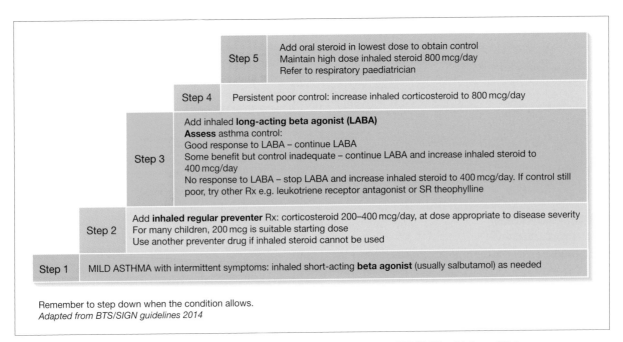

Figure 29.3 Stepwise management of asthma in children aged 5–12 years. Adapted from BTS/SIGN guidelines, 2014.

CASE

30 I'm worried about my memory

Joan Watts, age 81 years
Retired
PMH: hiatus hernia; laparoscopic cholecystectomy
Medication: omeprazole 20 mg daily

Joan and Harry Watts have been registered with you for many years. Both enjoy good health, by and large. You last saw Joan just over a year ago, although she did come to see the practice nurse more recently for her annual flu jab. Joan and Harry always attend together, and this is the case today. They both sit down in your consulting room, and you ask Joan what you can do for her today. Joan says, 'I'm worried about my memory.' You give Joan a little time to talk, and she describes how over the last year or so she finds it increasingly difficult to remember things. She gets stuck with names and dates, and often forgets what she has gone into a room to do. She says, 'I'm really worried about this, doctor.'

What would you like to ask next?

You have two options. One is to find out more about what she's worried about, the second is to explore the memory loss. You elect to ask her next, 'What are you worried about, Joan?'

Joan goes on to say that she is worried that she might be getting dementia. She's read about it in the papers, and she had a friend who had it. She's worried she'll end up like them and be a drain on Harry.

You decide to explore the memory loss more. What would you like to ask?

You could ask the following questions.
• 'Is there **anything** else you are struggling with?' Disorientation, getting lost and trouble understanding are all features of dementia.
• 'How has your **mood** been?' Stress and depression can both affect memory.
• 'Have there been any other **physical symptoms**, such as difficulty moving?' Some neurological disorders can present with dementia, e.g. Parkinson's.
• 'How is this affecting your life?' It's crucial to assess the **impact** on her life and Harry's.
• 'Are you **driving**? How is this?' There may be safety issues here.
These questions allow you to explore some of the key features of dementia. Note the questions are quite open, and give your patient an opportunity to expand and fill in the details.

Open and closed questions

Open questions are useful at the beginning of your history taking. They give the patient space to give you the important information. See the question above, how is this affecting your life. This question enables the patient to talk about any areas of her life that might be affected, such as her friendships, her ability to do the cooking, her ability to get about, etc.

Closed questions are useful when you are keen on being clear about a specific detail. In general this is useful later in your history taking. For instance you might want to clarify a particular diagnosis (e.g. what is the character of the chest pain), exclude a red flag (e.g. how long have you been passing blood in your stool) or explore a specific area of safety – in this case you are asking specifically about her driving.

Using mostly open questions, and then moving to a handful of appropriate closed questions helps GPs gain lots of information in a time-efficient way.

Tip
When you are next sitting in with a GP look out for when they ask open and closed questions.

Joan tells you that she's been struggling with shopping. She's been dong this for years, but she's been forgetting what to buy, or forgetting her list or her money. She has found this upsetting. She has never driven.

You should also find out about her behaviour. How would you best do this?

It is reasonable to explore this with Joan, simply asking about how her behaviour has been. You should also bring in Harry here. Joan doesn't have much to add, but Harry goes on to tell you that Joan hasn't always been herself this last year. She has been much more suspicious than she used to be, especially at night-time. She doesn't like it if he pops out to the shops, and can end up questioning him at length about his movements when he gets back.

Features of dementia

Impaired cognition:
• memory problems
• poor understanding of communication
• disorientation.
Change in behaviour:
• withdrawal
• depression, anxiety, agitation
• fearfulness, suspicion
• restlessness
• blunted affect
• poor sleep.
Struggling with activities of daily living:
• getting lost
• struggling with medication
• self-neglect
• struggling with shopping or cooking
• leaving things on in the house.
If occurring in the context of a neurological condition there may be features such as gait disturbance.

General Practice Cases at a Glance, First Edition. Carol Cooper and Martin L Block. © 2017 John Wiley & Sons, Ltd. Published 2017 by John Wiley & Sons, Ltd.

What examination would you perform?

You should check her **pulse** and **BP** and perform a simple **memory assessment test**, such as the 6-CIT or GPCOG assessment. These are recognized dementia screening tools that involve asking the patient specific questions which lead to an overall score. This score indicates the likelihood of dementia.

The Six-Item Cognitive Impairment Test (6-CIT)

Ask: 'What year is it?'
Score 4 if incorrect.
Ask: 'What month is it?'
Score 3 if incorrect.
Say: 'Repeat after me: John / Smith / 42 / High Street / Bedford'
Ask: 'About what time is it?'
Score 3 if more than 1 hour wrong.
Ask: 'Count backwards from 20 to one.'
Score 2 if one mistake; score 4 if two or more mistakes.
Ask: 'Say the months of the year in reverse.'
Score 2 if one mistake; score 4 if two or more mistakes.
Ask: 'Repeat the address phrase requested earlier.'
Score 2 for each mistake; maximum score 10 for five mistakes.
A total score of 8 or more suggests dementia.

From cks.nice.org.uk/dementia

Recognized screening tools for dementia

- 6-CIT (6-item Cognitive Impairment Test).
- GPCOG (General Practitioner Assessment of Cognition). http://www.gpcog.com.au/
- Mini-Cog.
- MIS (Memory Impairment Screen).
- MMSE (Mini Mental State Examination).

Joan's BP is 135/68, her pulse is 78 and regular.
Her 6-CIT score is 14, which is suggestive of dementia.

What is the likely diagnosis?

It is likely that this is a first presentation of dementia, but this diagnosis should be made formally in a memory clinic. A CT scan may well be necessary to confirm the diagnosis. Joan will also need blood tests to further clarify the picture. An abnormality here could point to a possible cause for dementia.

You tell Joan that the test you have done does show that she has some memory impairment, and a likely diagnosis is dementia. You explain that this is a condition where the brain works less powerfully and leads to problems with memory and thought processes. You explain there is a variety of possible causes, and that you will arrange for tests to be done immediately to investigate further, prior to getting her seen in a specialist clinic to confirm the diagnosis.

What tests should you arrange?

You should arrange the tests given in the box: GP investigations in dementia, including bloods, urinalysis and, if there are respiratory symptoms, a chest x-ray.

GP investigations in dementia

- Full blood count.
- U+E.
- Calcium.
- LFTs.
- TFTs.
- HBa1c.
- B12 and folate levels.

  Consider also:
- HIV and syphilis serology.
- MSU.
- CXR or ECG if respiratory or cardiovascular disease suspected.
- CT head will be performed in clinic.

You arrange the blood tests and book Joan in for a review appointment in three weeks. As you explain to Joan, when the results are back then it is likely that you will be referring her to the memory clinic to confirm whether or not the diagnosis is dementia.

Joan and Harry thank you for your time today. You see that Harry has a tear in his eye as they are leaving.

Management points

Some issues should be raised proactively during the course of the illness.
- Memory medications, such as donepezil (prescribed in memory clinic depending on results of tests).
- Dementia nurse support (e.g. for practical hints and tips and general support).
- Carers' support for Harry.
- Home carers (through social services).
- Legal issues (such as power of attorney, will, advanced directive). There is lots of useful information on the Age UK website.
- Dosette box for medication.

Resources

Age UK charity.
  www.ageuk.org.uk
CKS/NICE Dementia.
  www.cks.nice.org.uk/dementia

31 I've got this pain in my chest, Doctor

Karim Maliq, age 58 years

Taxi driver

PMH: type 2 diabetes; hypertension; acid reflux

Non-smoker

Medication: metformin 1 g bd, gliclazide 80 mg od, simvastatin 40 mg od, ramipril 10 mg od, omeprazole 20 mg od

Investigations: Hba1c 74 mmol/mol (8.9%), cholesterol 4.8 mmol/L

Mr Maliq attends today with his wife in an emergency appointment. He is of South Asian origin (Pakistan) but has lived in the UK for the last 18 years. He is a gentleman who you have seen over the past three years since he registered with the practice, who you have struggled to engage in treatment. His Hba1c was last checked a year ago and was 8.9. At this point you added in gliclazide to his treatment and had planned to follow him up after three months with a repeat Hba1c. This follow-up did not happen and this is the first time you have seen him since.

You welcome him into your room and ask him, 'What can I do for you today?'

Mr Maliq tells you he is very worried about a chest pain he has been experiencing since last night. He woke up with it at around 5am and felt unwell. His wife wanted him to call an ambulance but he wanted to wait to see you in the morning.

What questions do you want to ask about the chest pain?

You need to get a clear picture of the pain itself. An open question such as 'Tell me more about the pain' would be a good start. It is likely that Mr Maliq will give you lots of the important information without too much prompting, however it is important that you follow this up with some clear closed questions to complete the picture. SOCRATES is a good *aide mémoire* here.

SOCRATES pain assessment

Site – Where is the pain?
Onset – When did the pain start, and was it sudden or gradual?
Character – What does the pain feel like?
Radiation – Does the pain move anywhere?
Associations – Are there any other associated symptoms?
Time course – Does the pain follow any pattern?
Exacerbating/relieving factors – Does anything change the pain?
Severity – How bad is the pain? On a scale of 1–10?

It is useful to find out if he has had any previous episodes of pain prior to this episode.

Mr Maliq describes a pain that woke him up at 5am. The pain was a heavy central crushing chest pain which radiated into his left shoulder. He felt sweaty initially but this has now passed. The pain improved after about an hour from around 9/10 to 4/10, which is the pain level now. He tried Gaviscon but this did not help. The pain has persisted at a lower level throughout the morning, with the same 'heavy' character.

What is the most likely diagnosis here?

Mr Maliq's pain is most likely due to ischaemic heart disease, either a myocardial Infarction or unstable angina

What features in the history are suggestive of ischaemic heart disease?

- Site – central chest.
- Onset – sudden.
- Character – heavy, crushing.
- Radiation – into left shoulder (but note this is not always the case).
- Associations – sweating.
- Severity – the severity of the pain would point to an MI.
Risk factors: type 2 diabetes, hypertension.

Risk factors for ischaemic heart disease

- Smoking.
- Type 2 diabetes.
- Hypertension.
- High cholesterol.
- Family history.
- Obesity.

What examination would you perform?

You need to examine his **cardiovascular** and his **respiratory** system. It would be useful also to check his **oxygen saturations**.

His heart sounds are normal. His heart rate is regular at 68 bpm and there are no added sounds or murmurs. His BP is 114/76. His chest is clear and his oxygen sats are 98% on air.

Does the normal cardiovascular examination go against your working diagnosis of IHD?

No. Although it is reassuring that he is not in an abnormal rhythm, a normal cardiovascular examination is quite common in IHD.

What is your immediate management of this patient?

This gentleman has an **acute presentation of IHD**, likely to be MI, so should be treated as a medical emergency.

You should arrange for an immediate blue light ambulance to take him to hospital. He should have 300 mg aspirin (record this in your letter). You should also give some pain relief, such as a GTN spray and/or opiate analgesia, e.g. a slow iv administration of diamorphine 2.5–5 mg.

During this it is really important to keep Mr Maliq informed about what is going on. You need to give him a clear explanation of his suspected diagnosis and why you are taking it seriously.

General Practice Cases at a Glance, First Edition. Carol Cooper and Martin L Block. © 2017 John Wiley & Sons, Ltd. Published 2017 by John Wiley & Sons, Ltd.

What happens when you ring for an emergency ambulance?

The practice will have on its system the emergency contact number for the local ambulance services. If you can't find this number it's OK to dial 999.

The call operator will take you through some essential details (e.g. patient name and location) and will ask you some questions to ascertain the level of emergency and whether this represents an immediate threat to life. This would be the case with Mr Maliq, and as such a 'blue light' ambulance will be arranged. The operator will give you a reference number for the patient, which you should record in his records.

Should you give oxygen?

No, if the oxygen saturation is >94%, oxygen should not be given.

An ambulance arrives after 7 minutes and the paramedics help Mr Maliq into a wheelchair and take him with his wife to the nearest A+E.

You receive a letter from the hospital confirming your suspicion. Mr Maliq did have an MI and was treated acutely with angioplasty and stenting.

A few days after his discharge, Mrs Maliq drops in a card to the practice thanking you for your swift attention and for saving her husband's life.

Was there a missed opportunity?

It is unfortunate that Mr Maliq's Hba1c control has been poor and that he has not been attending follow-up. This case is a reminder of the importance of this (as his raised Hba1c would have increased his chance of having an MI), and a challenge in thinking about:

• How to educate and inform patients about the importance of control and follow-up. Of paramount importance here is the patient's understanding of their condition, and of the expected benefits of treatment. A patient will only follow a plan if they understand it and have ownership of it. Think also about when to bring the patient's family in to the discussion.

• The systems put in place to pick up and recall patients who fall away from follow-up.

Resources

Chest pain of recent onset: assessment and diagnosis (NICE, 2010).
    https://www.nice.org.uk/guidance/cg95/chapter/guidance

I've been having terrible stomach cramps

Jennifer Riley, age 31 years
Solicitor
PMH: nil of note
Medication: nil

Ms Riley is a newly registered patient at your practice and this is her first attendance. You can see from her records that she must have recently moved into the area. She is smartly dressed and walks confidently down the corridor to take a seat in your consulting room.

You ask her what you can do to help her.

Ms Riley explains that for several years she has been suffering from stomach cramps. She first experienced them what she was at university and they have continued on and off since then. She has noticed that she is much more likely to get these cramps when she is under stress or run down. She explains that she moved into town four months ago to start a new job. It's been pretty hectic since then, and her symptoms have flared up. Now they're as bad as they have ever been. She goes on to say that she has been a little constipated on and off over the past few months, but throughout this time she has also had some bouts of diarrhoea. In the past she has seen her GP from back home about this, but has never really been given a clear diagnosis.

What are your first thoughts on the diagnosis?

The most likely diagnosis here is irritable bowel syndrome (IBS).

Irritable bowel syndrome

Chronic, relapsing disorder of gastrointestinal function characterized by:
• abdominal pain or discomfort associated with, or relieved by, defecation
• change in bowel habit (constipation, diarrhoea or both)
• abdominal bloating.
The exact cause is unknown, but is probably multifactorial, with underlying:
• abnormal autonomic activity, central nervous system modulation and gastrointestinal motility
• visceral hypersensitivity
• abnormal gastrointestinal immune function.
From CKS NICE – IBS

You decide to explore the history further to rule out other possibilities.

What other conditions are in your differential diagnosis?

Differential diagnosis for IBS

Inflammatory bowel disease (e.g. Crohn's or UC).
Malignancy (bowel or ovarian).

Other causes of diarrhoea:
• coeliac disease
• infection.
Other causes of constipation:
• drug induced
• hypothyroidism.
Other causes of pain:
• peptic ulcer disease or reflux
• gallstones
• diverticular disease.

What questions might you ask to further clarify the diagnosis?

• 'Do you have any **other symptoms**?' This might give you important clues.
• 'Have you had any ► **bleeding**?'
• 'Any **weight loss**?' ► Weight loss or ► bleeding PR should always be taken seriously.
• Find out more about the pain. Where is it? What brings it on? What is it like?
• What **triggers** the symptoms? Are there any dietary triggers?
• What is her level of **exercise/activity**? IBS tends to be worse if this is low.

Ms Riley goes on to explain that the pain is cramping in nature and is also associated with bloating. It can be at any time of the day, but tends to be really bad before she passes her stool. This makes the pain a little better. The cramping tends to be all over her abdomen. There is never any blood in her stool and no weight loss.

Any more thoughts on the diagnosis?

IBS is still the most likely diagnosis. The history doesn't suggest malignancy, and your patient's answers fit your initial thoughts.

Features suggestive of malignancy

Bowel
► Unintentional and unexplained weight loss.
► Rectal bleeding.
► A change in bowel habit to looser or more frequent stools, persisting for more than 6 weeks, in a person over 60 years of age.
► Abdominal or rectal mass.
► Anaemia (Hb <10 g/100 mL in non-menstruating women, <11 g/100 mL in men).

Ovarian
► New-onset pelvic bloating (especially in women over 40).

Either
► A family history of bowel or ovarian cancer.

As well as assessing the likely diagnosis, get a sense of the impact the condition is having on her.

What question might you ask here?

Ask something simple and open like, 'What effect is this having on your life?'

Ms Riley says that so far she has been able to keep functioning in spite of the pain, but she had a day off a couple of weeks ago with it, and she feels that she is not able to do her best at work when she is having cramps. She also had to rush out of an important meeting recently to go to the toilet, which was really embarrassing.

You examine Ms Riley's abdomen. It is soft and diffusely bloated with patchy discomfort and mild tenderness throughout. There are no masses and there is no guarding.

What investigations should you do and why?

Bloods:
• full blood count, ESR or CRP – to help rule out inflammatory bowel disease
• coeliac antibody screen – to rule out coeliac disease.
An **ultrasound** scan could be done if you were considering gallstones or ovarian pathology. In this case it is not necessary.

You tell Ms Riley that you suspect that she has IBS, but you would like to do some simple blood tests to help rule out other possibilities. You arrange to see her with the results of the tests and give her a patient information leaflet on IBS to take away.

You see Ms Riley again and her blood results show a normal FBC and coeliac screen. Her ESR is 4 and her CRP is 1.

At this point it is important to give a clear positive diagnosis of IBS. How would you explain this?

Stick with a clear, jargon-free explanation like, 'From what you have told me, my examination and the blood tests, everything points to a diagnosis of irritable bowel syndrome or IBS. We don't know the exact cause of IBS, but it causes the bowel to become sensitive and uncomfortable. This can be made worse by stress and certain foods. Although we can't cure IBS there are lots of things that can be done to improve the condition.'

Patient information leaflets can be really useful here. Ms Riley has read the sheet you have given her, and also had a good look at some of the web resources highlighted, and agrees that this seems to make a lot of sense.

What management options should you discuss?

Lifestyle modifications

• Stress: identify stress and try to find time and ways to relax.
• Diet:
  • regular (unrushed) meals
  • regular (non-caffeine) drinks – 8 cups a day
  • limit fresh fruit to three portions a day
  • limit intake of insoluble fibre (e.g. bran-based cereals, wholemeal bread and rice), soluble fibre (e.g. oats) is better
  • consider referring to a dietician if no response to above; if diet is a major factor, consider exclusion diets.
• Exercise: increase physical activity level if this is low.

Medication (for symptom control)

• For pain/cramping: antispasmodic (e.g. mebeverine, peppermint oil).
• For constipation: bulk-forming laxative (e.g. ispaghula).
• For diarrhoea: anti-motility drug (e.g. loperamide).
If no response to the above consider a low-dose tricyclic antidepressant or SSRI.

Counselling/CBT

Consider if strong psychological factors.

You discuss these options with Ms Riley, with the aid of the patient information leaflet that you printed out last time. She was interested to read about lifestyle modification, and is already making some changes. She has also decided to get back into yoga, as she found it really helpful in decreasing her stress level in the past. She is keen to avoid medication if at all possible. She leaves the room with a clear diagnosis and a plan of what she can do to help things. She is also happy that there are no signs of anything potentially serious going on. She tells you that she will come back and see you if things don't improve.

Resources
CKS/NICE guidance: Irritable bowel syndrome.
    http://cks.nice.org.uk/irritable-bowel-syndrome

CASE

33 I'm concerned this mole has been growing

Anna Joseph, age 44 years
GP
PMH: appendicectomy aged 10; nil else of note
Medication: nil

Dr Joseph has booked to see you. Originally from Australia, she has lived and worked in the UK for the last eight years. She is a local GP and also a GP trainer. She and her young family have been registered with you for many years. You see her two daughters every now and again for routine childhood illnesses. Dr Joseph herself rarely comes to the GP, and is fit and well.

You welcome Dr Joseph to your room and ask her what you can do for her. She tells you that she is concerned about a mole on her forearm. She has had this mole for many years but recently things have changed; it has been growing a little and has become a little itchy. She is concerned that it may be a melanoma and thinks that it may need to be seen urgently. She tells you that she has lots of moles and freckles and is someone who burns easily.

What are the risk factors for malignant melanoma? Name at least three.

There are several risk factors for melanoma.

Dr Joseph is fair skinned, burns easily and grew up getting lots of sun exposure in Melbourne. She tells you that she would often get sunburnt in the summer, along with her sister. Nobody in her family have any history of skin cancers. She is aware she is at higher risk for melanoma, and that has influenced her decision to come and see you today.

Factors increasing the risk of melanoma

Skin lesions, such as:
• a high density of freckles or a tendency to freckle in the sun
• a large number of normal moles (risk increases with increasing number)
• five or more atypical moles.
Pale skin (type I and II) that burns easily; light-coloured eyes; red or light hair.
Unusually high sun exposure, particularly blistering sunburn.
Increasing age.
Female sex.
From CKS NICE Melanoma and Pigmented Lesions

What will you be looking for in your examination?

Your examination should cover two areas:
• a general assessment of Dr Joseph's skin
• the mole in question.
If Dr Joseph has numerous other moles and freckles, this will increase your level of suspicion. When you are assessing the mole

in question you should refer to the major and minor criteria listed in the referral guidelines for suspected cancer (see box). This helpful scoring system will guide you as to the likelihood of this mole being a melanoma. If the score is 3 or above, she should be referred under the urgent cancer pathway.

Suspected malignant melanoma – scoring criteria

Major features – score 2 points each:
• change in size
• irregular shape
• irregular colour.
Minor features – score 1 point each:
• largest diameter 7 mm or more
• inflammation
• oozing
• change in sensation.
Total score of 3 or more – **urgent referral.**
From NICE referral guidelines for suspected skin cancer

You examine Dr Joseph. She is skin type 1, and has numerous moles and freckles. The mole in question is 10 mm in diameter (she reports that it was formerly about 6–7 mm), is regular in shape but irregular in colour. It is not inflamed but she reports that it is itchy.

See Figures 33.1 and 33.2. Note the 'stuck on' appearance of the seborrhoeic keratosis. This is a common benign skin lesion.

What is her score and what should you do next?

You should use the scoring criteria above. In the case of Dr Joseph:
Major features:
• change in size – 2 points
• irregular in colour – 2 points.
Minor features:
• largest diameter 7 mm or more – 1 point
• change in sensation – 1 point.

Total – **6 points**

She also has several risk factors that further raise your level of suspicion.

Given her score (of 3 or greater) she requires an urgent assessment, and should be seen within two weeks in a specialist clinic.

What do you do next in the consultation?

This is the time for an explanation before going on to agree your management plan.

What you would like to cover in your explanation?

You should be clear that her mole has several features that increase the chance of it being a melanoma (were Dr Joseph not medically trained it would be important to be clear to your patient that a melanoma is a kind of skin cancer). Dr Joseph agrees with you. She was concerned that her mole may be a melanoma, and though she

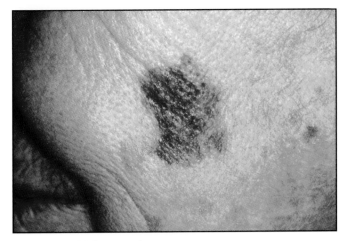

Figure 33.1 Malignant melanoma.

Source: National Cancer Institute. https://commons.wikimedia.org/wiki/
File:Melanoma_with_diameter_change.jpg. Public domain.

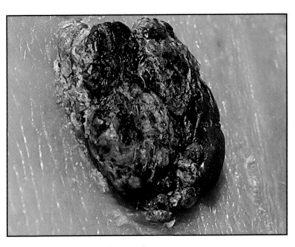

Figure 33.2 Seborrhoeic keratosis.

Source: Lmbuga https://commons.wikimedia.org/wiki/File:Queratose_
seborreica_1.jpg. Public domain.

'never comes to see the doctor' she knew that this was something that she needed to take seriously.

What should happen next?

Dr Joseph needs to be seen under the urgent cancer pathway, and you should send a referral to the 'two-week rule' clinic without delay.

When making an urgent cancer referral you should:
* act promptly
* check with the patient that their contact details are correct
* explain that they will be seen in two weeks
* be clear that you are referring as you are suspecting cancer.

You explain this clearly, and Dr Joseph knows exactly what to expect. You make the referral and Dr Joseph is seen the following week in the local dermatology clinic.

You subsequently receive correspondence that validates your level of suspicion. Dr Joseph is booked in to have the mole removed urgently. Further correspondence shows how Dr Joseph has a stage 1a melanoma (less than 1 mm in thickness with no evidence of spread). The melanoma was removed fully surgically. As such the prognosis is very good.

Dr Joseph sends you a card a few weeks later saying how she is grateful for your help and professionalism.

What do you need to consider in the future?

Next time you see Dr Joseph it is worth talking with her about:
* her increased risk of future melanoma
* what she can do to decrease this risk.

It is likely Dr Joseph is aware of these herself, but it would be worth encouraging her to cover up in the sun and to come back to see you if she has any other moles that develop any serious features.

Resources

CKS/NICE guidance: Melanoma and pigmented lesions.
   http://cks.nice.org.uk/melanoma-and-pigmented-lesions
NICE guidance: Referral guidelines for suspected cancer.
   http://www.nice.org.uk/guidance/cg27

CASE

34 I seem to have lost weight

Rashid Fawzy, age 43 years
TV engineer
PMH: peptic ulcer
Medication: nil

Rashid Fawzy hasn't attended the surgery for three years. Today he tells you he's been losing weight. He's not sure how much, or how long it's been going on, but his jeans are a lot looser than they used to be. He has always been slim and doesn't want to lose much more. He adds that he feels OK.

What useful questions might you ask? Write down at least five.

• 'Have you any **other symptoms**?' He has said he feels all right, but you may need to draw him out with more specific questions about his eating habits, any change in his bowels, cough or fever.
• Always ask about **night sweats** if there's weight loss, chronic cough or tiredness.
• 'Have you **travelled** abroad lately?'
• 'How is your **mood?**' and 'Are you **sleeping** all right?' can help uncover depression.
• 'What else is happening in your life?' is a useful catch-all question which can yield a lot of information about a person's social life, occupation and worries.

Rashid isn't doing anything differently. His menu is the same as ever, and his bowels haven't changed. He lives with his wife and three children. About five months ago, they went to Egypt to visit family. Nobody was ill there. Generally he sleeps well, but now that you mention it there have been some night sweats. He thought it was due to the new duvet, but it doesn't make his wife sweat. He doesn't smoke and has no cough.

While he talks, you find a previous weight in the records. Four years ago, Rashid weighed 73 kg. You weigh him now and he is 65 kg.

What is your impression so far?

There aren't many clues but he has lost over 10% of his body weight.

▶ Unintentional weight loss is a very significant symptom.
▶ Any symptom increases in significance in patients who consult infrequently.

The possibilities range across the whole of medicine and you now need to examine him to help determine the cause of his weight loss.

Some causes of weight loss

Reduced intake or absorption
• Oral thrush.
• Badly fitting dentures.
• Dysphagia.
• Anorexia.
• Food intolerance.
• Coeliac disease.

Infection
• TB.
• HIV.
• Parasitic infection.
• Brucellosis, Lyme disease and other infections.
• Bacterial endocarditis.

Mental health
• Depression or anxiety.

Endocrine and metabolic
• Hyperthyroidism.
• Diabetes (type 1).
• Addison's disease.
• Renal disease.
• Pancreatic disease.

Chronic disease
• Inflammatory arthritis or autoimmune disease, e.g. polymyositis.
• Parkinson's.
• Inflammatory bowel disease (e.g. ulcerative colitis, Crohn's).

Neoplastic
• Cancer.
• Lymphoma.
• Leukaemia.
• Carcinoid syndrome.

What do you particularly need to check in your examination?

• **Hands** can provide important clues: clubbing, splinter haemorrhages, koilonychia, tremor, sweating, and of course the pulse at the wrist.
• **Chest** (even though you may be requesting CXR shortly).
• **Abdomen** for masses or tenderness.
• **Lymph nodes** for any enlargement.
• You may also want to examine his **scrotum** for testicular lumps – remember to offer a chaperone.

Rashid declines a chaperone. On examination, his palms are a bit sweaty. While examining his abdomen, you notice a lump in the left groin. It is not a hernia. Rashid tells you he's had it a little while, maybe two or three months, though it has fluctuated in size. It is now a bit bigger than it was, he says. It is a firm tender lump about 3–4 cm in diameter, and feels like a lymph node.

You are surprised that Rashid didn't consult about this lump before, but he may have thought it was trivial as its size varied. Or he may have suspected it was serious and was afraid to know more.

What do you do now?

First finish the examination. Look for other lymph nodes, especially in the neck, axillae and supraclavicular fossae. Check for spleen and liver enlargement. It is still worth examining the testes (the lymphatic drainage of the testes is to the para-aortic nodes, not the inguinal region, but a thorough examination is helpful).

General Practice Cases at a Glance, First Edition. Carol Cooper and Martin L Block. © 2017 John Wiley & Sons, Ltd. Published 2017 by John Wiley & Sons, Ltd.

You find no other lymph nodes or masses, and his liver and spleen are normal.

Now what do you do?

He has unexplained lymph node enlargement and systemic symptoms (weight loss and night sweats).

According to NICE guidance, combinations of these signs/symptoms suggest haematological malignancy (this includes lymphoma):

- fatigue
- night sweats or fever
- weight loss
- itching
- breathlessness
- bruising
- bleeding
- recurrent infection
- bony pain
- alcohol-induced pain
- enlarged lymph nodes
- abdominal pain
- splenomegaly.

When you ask about alcohol-induced pain, Rashid says that as a Muslim he does not drink.

With the guideline in mind, you should refer Rashid to haematology urgently, or begin investigations and review him again very soon, with a view to urgent or fast-track referral.

You do not feel confident about the work-up and decide to refer him, having arranged a few tests which should be available when he is seen in the haematology clinic.

What do you tell Rashid?

As so often, it's a question of saying it might be grave without scaring the patient senseless. You can tell him something like, 'I'm concerned that this could be a serious blood or lymph condition, in which case the sooner it's diagnosed and treated, the better. It may not be anything much, but it still should to be taken seriously until the specialist has seen you.'

What tests do you request? And what may they reveal in lymphoma?

- CXR – widened mediastinum in mediastinal involvement.
- FBC – can be normal in lymphoma, or may show normochromic normocytic anaemia, pancytopenia, eosinophilia, neutrophilia, thrombocytosis or monocytosis.
- CRP/ESR – may be high.
- U&E/creatinine – may be abnormal and can influence treatment.
- LFTs – may be abnormal if the liver is involved.
- LDH – may indicate sarcoid or lymphoma (not a good tumour marker but can be used to follow up).
- Uric acid – can be raised in some forms of non-Hodgkin's lymphoma.
- HIV – useful in investigating weight loss, and a risk factor for lymphoma.
- Hepatitis B and C serology – useful in investigating weight loss, and a risk factor for lymphoma.

Lymphoma

The **fifth most common cancer** in the UK, and the most common cancer in teens and young adults.

Early diagnosis and treatment enable the best outcomes.

But a **huge challenge for GPs**:

- numbers are rising
- hard to diagnose because of the wide range of possible symptoms, often vague or non-specific
- two peaks of age distribution – young adult and older adult
- investigations can be inconclusive.

Two main types

Hodgkin's (HL) and non-Hodgkin's lymphoma (NHL), and many subtypes. NHL is about five times more common than HL. Over half of lymphomas in younger people are NHL. HL is more common in white races.

Classic presentation of HL is painless lymph node enlargement, but it can also be **painful and/or tender**.

► So-called '**B symptoms**' (night sweats, recurring fever >38 °C, weight loss >10% over 6 months) occur in 25% of lymphomas and are linked with advanced disease (i.e. spread) and with high-grade lymphoma.

► **Alcohol-induced pain** at site of node involvement is rare (up to 10% of patients) but is very specific for lymphoma.

Treatment

May be chemotherapy, or sometimes radiotherapy or even surgery if there are symptoms of compression. Monoclonal antibody treatments and biological therapies are also used for some types of lymphoma.

Prognosis

- NHL >50% survive 10 years or more.
- HL >80% survive 5 years or more.

Risk factors for lymphoma

- *Helicobacter pylori.*
- Hepatitis B and C.
- HIV.
- EB virus (in Burkitt's lymphoma).
- Smoking.
- Chronic inflammation.
- Organ transplantation and immune suppression.
- Crohn's disease.
- Family history of NHL or other haematological malignancy.

Rashid is found to have high-grade NHL, and receives chemotherapy. The practice is asked to vaccinate him against *Pneumococcus* (polyvalent vaccine), flu, Hib and meningitis C (Men C conjugate vaccine).

Resources

CKS Haematological malignancy – suspected.
http://cks.nice.org.uk/haematological-malignancy-suspected#!scenario

Lymphoma Association (charity) info for patients and families; e-learning module for GPs.
http://www.lymphomas.org.uk/

CASE

35 I'm worried about my erection

> **Ray Walters, age 54 years**
> Bus driver
> PMH: nil of note
> Medication: nil

Mr Walters has been registered at the practice for about 30 years but has not been seen in the last eight years, and that was for a bout of otitis media. He looks a bit embarrassed as he sits down. You smile, hoping to put him at ease. You start out by asking him what you can do to help him today. Mr Walters says, 'It's quite personal, doctor. You know I'm not one to trouble you, but…I'm worried about my erection.'

What should you do next?

At this point you should still give Mr Walters a little more time to talk. If you interrupt then you may miss out on some useful information that he needs to share with you. A simple nod and some open body language may be enough to encourage him to talk a little more.

Mr Walters hesitates for a second before continuing. 'It's not easy to talk about these things, you know. Anyway, I first noticed it about a year ago. My erection was less strong than it used to be. I thought it was just a part of getting older, but things got steadily worse. Most times I can hardly get an erection at all, and it's having an effect on my marriage. My wife is very understanding but I feel really guilty about it. I've heard about the Viagra and all that, but I thought I'd better go and see you, rather than buy something online. What can I do?'

You have learned quite a lot already. You now have a clear idea on the timeframe, the level of symptoms and the impact it is having on him. He also has a clear practical agenda: he is here to do something about his problem.

What specific areas should you ask about in your history?

- **Relationship** status.
- Present and previous erection quality (including **early morning** and masturbatory erections).
- Issues with sexual aversion or **pain** (including for his partner).
- **Lifestyle** factors (e.g. alcohol, smoking and drugs, including cannabis).
- Treatments already tried.
- Symptoms suggesting **hypogonadism**: reduced energy levels, loss of libido, loss of body hair or spontaneous hot flushes.

Mr Walters' embarrassment will ease if you conduct the consultation with a sympathetic and open manner. If you are not embarrassed then, as the consultation progresses, neither will he be. A questionnaire like the **IIEF** (International Index of Erectile Function, see Resources) can help if you or he find it difficult to discuss the full details.

Mr Walters tells you he has been married to his partner for over 30 years. His erection used to be fine, up until a year ago, when things started to deteriorate. He is an ex-smoker, having given up 10 years ago. He drinks a couple of beers on a Friday night but otherwise his alcohol intake is minimal. He has never taken any drugs. He hasn't tried anything yet. He has also noticed that his early morning erections are not happening and he struggles also to get an erection on masturbation.

Is this likely that the nature of the problem is physical or psychological?

The gradual progressive onset, his age and the absence of early morning and masturbatory erections all point to this being physical. Erection is dependent on arterial blood flow into the penis.

What are the main physical causes?

- **Vascular:** atherosclerosis affecting penile blood vessels has the same risk factors for cardiovascular disease (diabetes, hypertension, smoking, raised cholesterol, family history).
- **Neurological**: anything that effects the nerves to the penis, e.g. diabetes, stroke, MS, Parkinson's disease, spinal cord injury, radical prostatectomy.
- **Alcohol** and **drug** use (such as cannabis and heroin).
- **Medications** (e.g. antidepressants, betablockers, diuretics).
- **Hormonal** deficiency (low testosterone).

What examination should you do?

You should:
- check BP
- measure BMI
- check for signs of hypogonadism (such as small testes, loss of body hair, breast growth).

Mr Walters has no signs of hypogonadism, his BMI is 30.5 and his BP is 137/64.

What tests should you arrange?

You should arrange the following blood tests:
- Hba1c
- lipid profile (and use the information to calculate the 10-year cardiovascular risk)
- 9am testosterone level.

Tip

Erectile dysfunction is a marker for cardiovascular disease. Always calculate 10-year cardiovascular risk in patients presenting with ED. Through this you will pick up patients who are at higher risk of cardiovascular disease – and you will save lives.

Mr Walters books back in to see you to discuss the results and plan his treatment. His results show:
- a normal testosterone level
- total cholesterol 5.4 mmol/L
- Hba1c 8.8%.

What is the likely diagnosis?

Although the Hba1c needs repeating for confirmation, Mr Walters has a likely diagnosis of type 2 diabetes. This has probably been contributing to his erectile dysfunction through a combination of small vessel disease and local neurological damage.

Hba1c levels and diabetes

- Hba1c ≥48 mmol/mol (6.5%) on two occasions: diabetes.
- Hba1c 42–47 mmol/mol (6.0–6.4%) inclusive: pre-diabetes.
- Hba1c 41 mmol/mol (5.9%) or less: normal.

What should your management be?

There are two threads here: firstly manage his new diagnosis of diabetes (see Resources), and secondly manage his erectile dysfunction. It should improve with a combination of the following.

Lifestyle measures:
- stop smoking
- alcohol reduction
- weight loss
- regular exercise
- consider decreasing cycling if >3 hours a week (can affect penile nerve supply).

Medication:
- Phosphodiesterase-5 inhibitors (e.g. sildenafil).

Consider referral to clinic for **other treatments** (e.g. vacuum pumps, penile injection, penile implant) if PDE-5 inhibitors don't help.

Consider **psychological therapy** if ED is felt to be due to a psychological cause. A physical cause doesn't exclude anxiety and other psychological factors.

You discuss the above with Mr Walters, who agrees he would definitely benefit from weight reduction (his BMI is 30.5) and that regular exercise would help with this. He is motivated to do this, especially as it may also improve his diabetes. He is also keen to try a medication and you give him a prescription for sildenafil 50 mg to try. You advise him to return to see you in a month or two to let you know how he has got on.

What should you advise Mr Walters before starting sildenafil?

- Sildenafil takes at least 30 minutes before it is active.
- Sexual stimulation is still required to produce an erection.
- Common side effects include headache, flushing, blocked nose, dyspepsia, nausea and visual disturbance.
- It should be avoided if there is severe cardiovascular disease or a recent MI.

Mr Walters is grateful to you for taking his problem seriously and for your practical help and advice. He is hopeful things may improve with his lifestyle measures and sildenafil. You arrange a follow-up appointment in a couple of months time.

Resources

Patient. Advice and Information: Erectile dysfunction (impotence).
  http://www.patient.co.uk/health/erectile-dysfunction-impotence
CKS/NICE Erectile dysfunction.
  http://cks.nice.org.uk/erectile-dysfunction
CKS/NICE Diabetes.
  http://cks.nice.org.uk/diabetes-type-2
IEEF Questionnaire.
  http://www.camurology.org.uk/wp-content/uploads/interpretation-of-the-iief.pdf
You may also like to try Case 22: 'I've come for the results of my blood tests'.

CASE

36 I think the cancer has got me

Home visit

Alan Wright, age 58 years

Unemployed

PMH: Ca lung (adenocarcinoma) with likely hepatic secondaries; high cholesterol

Medication: paracetamol 1 g qds prn, movicol 2 sachets daily, atorvastatin 20 mg daily

---

Mr Wright was diagnosed with lung cancer two months ago. He presented with a persistent cough, haemoptysis and weight loss. He was referred under the 'two-week rule' to the suspected lung cancer clinic and, following a CT scan and bronchoscopy, he was diagnosed with adenocarcinoma of the lung.

The CT scan revealed widespread lymphatic spread and two masses in the liver, which were consistent with hepatic metastases. He was given a short course of palliative radiotherapy which has now finished. His care is shared between you and the local community palliative care team, who have been seeing him twice weekly. You are aiming to see him at least every two weeks for support and to keep an eye on his progress. Today is a scheduled home visit.

Mr Wright lives in a ground floor flat with his wife Sue. You call Sue before your visit to confirm you are leaving the practice and she tells you that things are not good with Alan. She is worried that he is going downhill fast.

You last saw Mr Wright two weeks ago, and you find his deterioration significant. He has lost weight and looks exhausted, lying in bed. You greet Mr Wright and sit down on a chair beside his bed. He thanks you for coming out to see him today. You ask him how he is doing. Mr Wright's first words are, 'I think the cancer has got me.' He sighs and shakes his head.

What should you approach in this consultation?

You don't need to ask lots of questions here. It's time to listen to what Mr Wright needs to say. Just give him some space to talk, and encouragement to carry on talking. Throughout this visit your role is to offer support, to show Mr Wright kindness and sympathy and to hear what he has to say. You offer Mr Wright a simple warm, 'I'm sorry to hear this,' and he carries on talking.

'Things are getting worse this week, I can't eat anything and I'm getting really tired if I do anything. I can hardly wash or clean myself. I can barely walk to the bathroom without having to sit down halfway. I think this is the end, doctor.'

What should you ask to find out more about symptoms?

Find out if there is anything that Mr Wright thinks you could help with.

- Is he in any **pain**?
- Are there any **other troubling symptoms** like nausea, diarrhoea, breathlessness or cough?

Mr Wright says that he does not have any other major symptoms. It's mainly weakness and loss of appetite. He did have a little

constipation last week, but his nurse advised he start some Movicol sachets. One of your colleagues prescribed these and he has found these helpful.

What other areas would you like to talk about today?

You should make time to talk about the following.

- **Support**: what level of support do they both have (e.g. any home carers)? Is this enough?
- **Plans** for what to do if there is any further deterioration.
- **Resuscitation** status.
- Intended **place of death**.

These can feel like difficult areas to talk about, but patients at the end of life often appreciate them being addressed by their doctor. Mrs Wright says that they have a carer come twice a day to help with washing and dressing. She is managing to keep on top of everything else. They have spoken to the palliative care nurse about plans for further deterioration and Mr Wright wants to die at home.

You should give Mr Wright the space and opportunity to talk openly about death.

Jane, the palliative care nurse, had warned you about Mr Wright's deterioration and you have come prepared to discuss resuscitation status. You have brought the appropriate form with you today.

How should you talk about resuscitation status with Mr Wright?

Your approach should be open, honest and clear. The discussion should be grounded in Mr Wright's (and his wife's) values and their understanding of his deterioration. You should then move on to find out what they would want to happen when things deteriorate further and his heart stops beating. Mr Wright is clear that he does not want any CPR and that he is prepared for his death. You complete the resuscitation status forms and leave the original copy in a clearly visible place, clipped to top of his nursing folder.

Mr Wright is grateful to you for discussing this openly with him and for your professionalism today and over the years. There isn't anything else he needs help with.

Have a look at his medications. Do they all need to continue?

Mr Wright should stop his statin, if he has not done so already, as it has no benefit at this point in his life.

Paracetamol (for pain) should be continued if needed. Movicol has helped his recent constipation and should be continued.

Mr Wright thanks you for popping over today and wishes you well. You return to the practice.

What should you do following your discussion with Mr Wright about his resuscitation status?

You should clearly record this in his medical record. It is likely that the area you work in has an electronic system for recording palliative care patient's care plan. This will be accessible to Ambulance Services and Out of Hours GP services. You update Mr Wright's record with his resuscitation status. The ambulance service will now be aware of this. You also drop Jane, the palliative care nurse, a quick email to update her on the outcome of your visit.

General Practice Cases at a Glance, First Edition. Carol Cooper and Martin L Block. © 2017 John Wiley & Sons, Ltd. Published 2017 by John Wiley & Sons, Ltd.

The following day you get a call from Mrs Wright to say her husband died last night in his sleep. She tells you the out of hours doctor visited in the night to confirm death. You offer her your condolences. She thanks you for your care of her husband. You receive a call from the coroner who asks you if you are happy to issue a death certificate.

Should you issue a death certificate?

Yes. You have seen Mr Wright within the last two weeks and this is an expected death. You can feel confident of the cause of death.

Key point

A death certificate may be issued by a doctor who has provided care during the last illness and who has seen the deceased within 14 days of death (28 days in Northern Ireland) or after death. They should be confident about the cause of death.

What should you record as the cause of death on the death certificate?

You should complete the certificate as:

  1 (a) Metastatic Lung Cancer
  The other sections should remain unfilled.

Cause of death the disease or condition thought to be the underlying cause should appear in the lowest completed line of part I

I	(a) Disease or condition leading directly to death	
	(b) other disease or condition, if any, leading to I(a)	
	(c) other disease or condition, if any, leading to I(b)	
II	Other significant conditions contributing to death but not related to the disease or condition causing it	

Figure 36.1 Death certificate.

Resources

Government guidance on how to complete a death certificate.
  http://www.gro.gov.uk/images/medcert_July_2010.pdf
Cancer research UK.
  http://www.cancerresearchuk.org/

37 I'm all over the place these days

Thomas Graham, age 46 years

Builder and decorator
PMH: elbow injury; traumatic amputation of L little finger
Medication: nil

Thomas Graham attends with his wife Tracey and says he's feeling rough and 'all over the place'. Tracey adds that she's really concerned. It's been going on for ages and she hopes you can do something. From this vague beginning, you establish that he's worried all the time. 'He keeps thinking something terrible is going to happen,' says Tracey.

You try to get Mr Graham to speak for himself, but he says, 'She can explain it better.' It has been building up for about two years, since the elbow injury that kept him off work for four months. They have three children living at home. Tracey works as a cleaner in a supermarket.

The symptoms are imprecise but they point towards anxiety. Mr Graham isn't very talkative and you decide you must draw him out.

What useful questions might you ask him at this stage? Write down at least six.

- 'Are you worried about **something in particular**?' This might point towards a specific stressor, or a phobia.
- 'What makes you **better**? And what makes you **worse**?'
- 'Are you able **to work** at the moment?'
- 'What do you think the trouble is?' and 'What do you hope I'll be able to do for you?' While Mr Graham may not be articulate or educated, every patient deserves to air his **ideas, concerns and expectations**.
- 'Do you get out of breath? What about pins and needles?' These are possible symptoms of **panic attack**.
- 'Do you have any other symptoms?' This could point to **physical disease**, or reveal anxieties about disease.
- 'Have you had any **mental health problems in the past**?'
- 'Do you drink **alcohol**? Are you taking any **drugs of any kind**?' Make sure you ask about street drugs. You may need to ask some of the more sensitive questions again when his wife isn't present.

As you speak, you assess his mental state from his demeanour. He is thin, dishevelled and fidgety. His speech seems hesitant, and he looks at the floor, avoiding eye contact.

He tells you he's always worried about something, mainly a disaster like having an injury or becoming disabled so that he can't earn money. He is currently working. Night-time is worst, and nothing makes him better except for a couple of beers. He is a smoker, and drinks 'the normal amount', which you discover is around three pints a day, more at weekends. He does not take any drugs. His heart races sometimes. Three times he's had attacks in the night when he struggled to breathe and got pins and needles. There are no obvious triggers and he doesn't know what the problem is. He hopes you can sort him out. A relative in Ireland got really bad and the doctor gave him Valium.

His fear of injury at work is not wholly irrational, but his response to it seems exaggerated.

What do you say to his suggestion of some Valium (diazepam)?

Try something like, 'It wouldn't be a good thing for you right now as it can be habit-forming. I'm sure we can find another solution for you.' Do not criticize the doctor who prescribed them for his relative as you don't know the circumstances. As benzodiazepines are habit-forming, there are dangers in prescribing them for chronic conditions, though you might consider them for a short, well defined period or an event such as a flight for someone with fear of flying.

Anxiety disorders

Anxiety disorders are common and range from **generalized anxiety disorder** (GAD) to **panic disorder**. Around a quarter of adults will develop an anxiety disorder at some point, often between 35 and 55 years of age.

GAD affects around 5% of the population. There is typically uncontrollable, disproportionate and widespread worry. There may also be cognitive and behavioural symptoms, and/or somatic features including tiredness, insomnia, palpitations, headache and bowel disturbance. These can seriously impair daily life.

The origin of GAD is unknown but there may a genetic element. Chronic illness can lead to or co-exist with GAD. Depression can co-exist with GAD. GAD can lead to substance abuse, and vice versa.

GAD symptoms can be lifelong, but two thirds report mild or no impairment at six years. The outlook is often worse in those with physical illness and lower social class.

Management is best by a stepped-care approach. Co-morbidities like depression may need to be treated first.

1 For mild anxiety symptoms, especially if present less than six months, active monitoring. If the anxiety symptoms are mild and/or present for less than six months, active monitoring and patient education should be tried.

2 If symptoms do not resolve, try low-intensity psychological intervention, e.g. individual facilitated or non-facilitated self-help or psychoeducational group therapy.

3 If marked functional impairment, or symptoms have not resolved, **either** a high-intensity psychological intervention (e.g. applied relaxation or cognitive behavioural therapy), or drug therapy should be offered, depending on the patient's wishes. Drug therapy should be an SSRI, with sertraline the drug of choice (despite its use for GAD being off-label). If this isn't tolerated, try an SNRI or consider pregabalin.

4 Refer for specialist treatment if inadequate response to both elements of step 3, very marked functional impairment, complex GAD, or high risk of self-harm, self-neglect or suicide.

Panic disorder affects about 1% of the population, women more than men. Typically there is severe overwhelming anxiety, shortness of breath, palpitations, sweating, tremor, nausea and fear of dying. Patients may present to A&E.

General Practice Cases at a Glance, First Edition. Carol Cooper and Martin L Block. © 2017 John Wiley & Sons, Ltd. Published 2017 by John Wiley & Sons, Ltd.

Hyperventilation can occur: paroxysms of rapid breathing, feeling short of breath, often chest discomfort, dizziness, and numbness or tingling in fingers (and sometimes toes). There may be perioral tingling and carpopedal spasm (Trousseau's sign with main d'accoucheur).

Management of panic disorder is stepwise.

1 Recognition and correct diagnosis.

2 Management in primary care: psychological treatment (ideally CBT), medication (usualy SSRI) and self-help.

3 Review and consider other therapies.

4 Review and consider referral to specialist mental health services.

5 Care within specialist mental health services.

From CKS/NICE on generalized anxiety disorder

Is there anything you should rule out here? Write down two things.

- **Depression**, which can co-exist with anxiety and should be treated first.
- **Physical illnesses that can mimic anxiety**, notably hyperthyroidism, asthma and arrhythmia.

Mr Graham has no features of depression. He has not lost weight and has no bowel symptoms. However, he tells you he always has a bit of a cough, and he wants to know if his heart is OK.

You examine him at this point. His chest is clear, BP is 153/98 and PEFR is 450 (he says he is 5'11 1/2", which is 1.81 m).

Are you able to reassure him about his physical health?

No. He may have hypertension. He could also have COPD or some other respiratory problem. However today you can probably safely say that most of his symptoms are due to anxiety disorder, which is 'a form of worrying that gets out of control'.

You should arrange some tests, including ECG and FBC, U&E, LFTs, TFTs, lipids and fasting glucose. These could be done today, although there is a risk of making him more anxious. An alternative is to defer them until you review him in two weeks.

Meanwhile you can offer him printed or online patient information (see Resources). He may not be able to digest it all in one go, but his wife is involved and between them they should get some benefit from these sources.

Resources

Clinical Knowledge Summaries: Generalized anxiety disorder.
http://cks.nice.org.uk/generalized-anxiety-disorder#!topicsummary
NICE guideline CG113: Generalised anxiety disorder and panic disorder (with or without agoraphobia) in adults: Management in primary, secondary and community care.
http://www.nice.org.uk/guidance/cg113/
Includes information for patients.
http://www.nice.org.uk/guidance/cg113/ifp/chapter/generalised-anxiety-disorder-gad
Mind (charity): information for patients.
www.mind.org.uk
You may also like to try Case 44: 'Doctor, I'm just feeling really down.'

CASE

38 She's had tummy ache for two days

Aimee Wilkinson, age 7 years

Schoolgirl

PMH: neonatal jaundice; two episodes of otitis media

Medication: nil

Aimee Wilkinson is brought in by her mother. She has had 'tummy ache' for nearly two days and was sent home from school yesterday morning. Her immunizations are up to date and her only PMH is neonatal jaundice and two episodes of otitis media.

What useful questions might you ask? Write down at least five.

• 'What's the pain like?' You want to know if it's continuous, how bad it is, whether it's keeping her awake, as well as other features (think SOCRATES).

• 'Has she had it before?' Some 10% of schoolchildren have recurrent abdominal pain.

• 'Is there **diarrhoea** or **vomiting**?'

• 'Is she **constipated**?' Constipation is a common cause of abdominal pain, but a constipated child can also have a more serious cause for her pain.

• 'Does it hurt to **wee**?' However UTI does not always cause urinary symptoms in children.

• 'Has she had a **fever**?' This suggests an infective cause, though not necessarily intra-abdominal.

• 'Are there any illnesses in the **family**?' You should think of diabetes and inflammatory bowel disease, but a family history of migraine is also important.

• 'How are things generally?' An open question like this may reveal a new baby in the family or problems at school.

Some questions you can ask Aimee directly, but at this age it's best to start with questions to the parent, especially if the child doesn't know you. Use age-appropriate words like 'poo' ('motions' and 'constipation' are likely to baffle). Consider 'Does it hurt to poo?' and 'Do you have to sit on the toilet for a long time? Do you have to push hard? What do your poos look like?'

Aimee has had similar pain before, but not as bad. There are no urinary symptoms and she hasn't opened her bowels for two days. Her mother has occasional migraine. Aimee shrugs when you ask about school, but she smiles as she does so, and mother tells you she has lots of friends.

What do you look for when examining this child?

• Obviously examine the abdomen. It can help to ask first 'Can you point to where it hurts?' Make sure the child is comfortable being examined, and that you have the parent's consent as well. Note that a reluctant child still needs to be examined, possibly even more so than a compliant one as she is more likely to be unwell. Ask the child to suck in her tummy, and puff out and cough before palpating in order to assess for ▶ peritonism. Listen first. Your stethoscope can then be used to gently press again to assess for tenderness without the child's knowledge. Watch the child's face as you examine her abdomen.

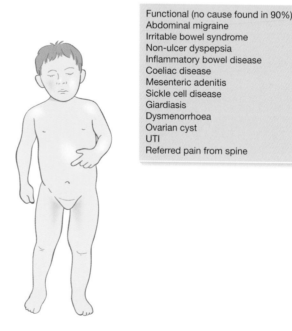

Causes of abdominal pain in children

Surgical:
Appendicitis
Meckel's diverticulitis
Intestinal obstruction
Intussusception
Obstructed or strangulated hernia
Pancreatitis (e.g. mumps)
Testicular torsion
Ovarian cyst (especially if it bleeds or undergoes torsion)

Medical:
Gastroenteritis
UTI
Tonsillitis/scarlet fever
Mesenteric adenitis
Henoch–Schönlein purpura
Sickle cell crisis
Diabetic keto-acidosis
Inflammatory bowel disease
Leukaemia
Lower lobe pneumonia
Referred pain from the spine
Rare causes such as nephroblastoma, neuroblastoma, hydatid cysts

Remember the possibility of ectopic pregnancy and/or pelvic inflammatory disease

Causes of recurrent abdominal pain

Functional (no cause found in 90%)
Abdominal migraine
Irritable bowel syndrome
Non-ulcer dyspepsia
Inflammatory bowel disease
Coeliac disease
Mesenteric adenitis
Sickle cell disease
Giardiasis
Dysmenorrhoea
Ovarian cyst
UTI
Referred pain from spine

Figure 38.1 Causes of abdominal pain in children.

General Practice Cases at a Glance, First Edition. Carol Cooper and Martin L Block. © 2017 John Wiley & Sons, Ltd. Published 2017 by John Wiley & Sons, Ltd.

- Take the **temperature**.
- Check the pulse and get an idea of her circulatory state. What's the capillary return, for instance?
- Look at the **tongue** and **throat**. There could be tonsillitis. In doing so, note the breath: is there a foetor (suggestive of appendicitis) or a ketotic smell? Linked with diabetic keto-acidosis, this smells of pear drops. Not all people can smell it.
- Feel for **lymph nodes** in the neck.
- Listen to the **chest** (she might have a lower lobe pneumonia).
- Note any **rashes** (Henoch–Schönlein purpura, scarlet fever, signs of systemic illness).
- Assess whether this child is of expected height and weight **for her age**. If you're not sure, measure.
- Finally ask yourself one vital question: **Is this child ill?**

Signs of peritoneal irritation

- Movement makes the pain worse.
- Pain on coughing.
- Guarding.
- Rigidity.
- Rebound.
- Percussion tenderness.

Aimee is a bit pale but does not look ill to you. Her temperature is normal and there are no rashes. Although she pointed to the area around her navel, she is only tender deep in both iliac fossae. Bowel sounds are normal. There is no peritoneal irritation (see box). Her throat and chest are normal, and her breath does not smell.

Key point

Whenever you see a child, always ask yourself 'Is this child ill?'

Should you do a rectal examination?

No. It is intrusive and unlikely to add anything to the diagnosis.

What are your thoughts at this stage? Write down three possibilities.

- Migraine.
- Functional pain.
- UTI.
- Diabetes (unlikely in such a well child, but it has not yet been excluded).

What do you do now?

- Test the urine with a dipstick.

Reassuringly, you find nothing amiss in the urine: no blood, protein, sugar, ketones or nitrites. This makes both UTI and diabetes unlikely. **However it still does not mean the pain is functional, due to migraine, or can safely be ignored.** Aimee could, for example, be developing appendicitis or Meckel's diverticulitis. There are also many rarer causes of abdominal pain. These are, by definition, much less likely, but they are often very serious. The GP is often the first port of call so you must know about them, and you must 'safety-net'.

It would be reasonable to tell Aimee and her mother that you suspect it's a type of migraine which is not unusual in children of her age. It's not a serious condition, but you'd like to see her again tomorrow or the next day, just to check. If things by any chance worsen before then, they should contact the practice.

Resources

Patient.co.uk.
http://www.patient.co.uk/doctor/abdominal-pain-in-children
Miall L, Rudolf M and Smith D. *Paediatrics at a Glance*. 3rd edn. Oxford: Wiley-Blackwell, 2012.

CASE

39

I don't want to have my period when I am on holiday

Farida El-Najjar, age 21 years
Accountancy student
PMH: acne
Medication: Dalacin T

Farida tells you she is going away in three weeks' time, and does not want to have a period while she is away. When you ask where she is going, you discover that her trip is a pilgrimage ('Hajj') to Mecca rather than a holiday. She has never taken the contraceptive pill.

What important questions do you ask her? Write down three.

• What is her **usual cycle**?
• Does she require **contraception**, or does she simply want to **avoid a period**? During the annual Hajj, it can be inconvenient to deal with a period, and a menstruating woman cannot perform all the rituals of Hajj. While you may deduce from your conversation so far that she is an observant Muslim, you should not assume this means she does not need contraception, so ask in a matter-of-fact, non-judgemental way.
• **When** is she going and for **how long**? Is it important for her to avoid a period during the entire absence? Hajj is normally at least 5 days, but the length of the trip depends on how she is getting there. Her period began 4 days ago and has just finished. It is usually regular, just about every 26–28 days. It is often heavy, and it is always painful for the first day or so. She tells you she is single and therefore does not need contraception. She and her family are flying to Saudi Arabia in a month and will be away about a week in all. She would prefer to delay the period for the whole trip until after she returns. This is her first trip to Mecca. She adds that a Muslim need only go once in his or her lifetime.

What are the two main treatment options here?

• **Norethisterone** is a progestogen licensed for postponement of menstruation. The usual dose is 5 mg tds beginning three days before the expected onset of a period. Tablets are often prescribed for up to 10–14 days. Bleeding normally starts two or three days after the drug is stopped.
• The **combined oral contraceptive pill** (COCP) can also be used to delay menstruation, though technically monthly bleeds on the Pill are withdrawal bleeds, not periods. Farida could start taking it on day five of the current cycle, which should be tomorrow (but always check what patients mean when they say they are on a particular day, as many of them count the first day of a period as day zero). If she takes two Pill packets consecutively without a break, she will avoid a bleed.

In Farida's case, is there one option you might suggest in preference to the other?

A COCP may be preferable to norethisterone, which is androgenic and could worsen her acne. Norethisterone is also linked with bloating, weight change, breast tenderness, nausea, and headache, but these can occur with the COCP too.

After the Hajj, she may wish to stay on it for dysmenorrhoea and heavy periods, though mefenamic acid is also an option which she has yet to try.

You must ensure that the Pill is acceptable to her. Emphasize that many girls and women take the Pill for reasons other than contraception. This is important not just for Farida's understanding, but in case any relatives jump to the wrong conclusion.

Once you tell Farida this, as well as the fact that norethisterone may 'stir up' her acne, she says she is happy to take the Pill. She is particularly pleased to know that the Pill often makes periods lighter and less painful, and would consider staying on it after her trip 'if it agrees with me'.

What questions should you ask to ensure the Pill is appropriate for her? Write down four of the most important points to cover.

• 'Have you ever had a **DVT** or blood clot in the legs or in the lungs?' And is there a family history of these?
• 'Do you **smoke**?' Observant Muslims do not smoke but it is good practice to ask anyway.
• 'Do you get **migraines**?' A history of migraine with aura raises the risk of stroke while on OCP by two- to four-fold.
• 'Have you ever been **jaundiced** or gone yellow?' Various forms of liver disease and gall bladder disease can contraindicate the OCP.
• 'Do you wear **contact lenses**?' This is not a contraindication, but contact lens wearers can find their lenses become uncomfortable on starting the Pill.

Even if Farida only takes the OCP for a couple of months, you must still ensure it is safe for her. There is a long list of potential contraindications.

UK Medical Eligibility Criteria (UKMEC) for the Oral Contraceptive

The UKMEC was initially produced in 2006, adapted from the World Health Organization (WHO) medical eligibility criteria, and then updated in 2009. Conditions are classified into four categories, with increasing risk to users of contraception:
Category 1: no restriction to use.
Category 2: advantages of use of the method of contraception generally outweigh the risks.
Category 3: risks generally outweigh advantages. Use not usually recommended.
Category 4: use of the contraceptive method would result in unacceptable risk to health.

What examination do you perform?

Take her **blood pressure**.
It is 126/88 and you tell her it is normal.

Now which type of COCP would you prescribe?

Prescribe a fixed-dose COCP, without dummy pills. Biphasic and triphasic Pills taken without a break will not prevent a withdrawal bleed. A woman would have to take the last phase of the pills from the second pack immediately after finishing the first pack.

General Practice Cases at a Glance, First Edition. Carol Cooper and Martin L Block. © 2017 John Wiley & Sons, Ltd. Published 2017 by John Wiley & Sons, Ltd.

You might also want to want to prescribe a Pill with one of the less androgenic progestogens: desogestrel, drospirenone, gestodene, norgestimate. However the first three are associated with a higher risk of VTE (venous thromboembolism) – see BNF.

You check the BNF and decide to go for a less androgenic Pill.

What might you prescribe?

Options include Marvelon, Mercilon, Yasmin, Femodene, Femodette, Millinette, Gedarel. However, if Farida opts for a short treatment duration of two months or so, the androgenicity may not matter and Microgynon or similar would be suitable.

Is there anything else you should do for Farida today?

The Hajj presents many health challenges, most of them a result of the huge crowds that gather. Two million people a year from all over the world go to Mecca (also known as Makkah) to perform Hajj. As a GP you should be aware of some of them so that you can direct patients appropriately.

Some health aspects of Hajj

Infections

Respiratory infections are the most common infections.

Vaccines needed

- Quadrivalent meningococcal (ACW135Y) vaccine is essential (carriage rates for meningococcus can be 80%).
- Up-to-date routine immunizations also needed.
- Consider flu vaccine especially for high-risk patients.
- Consider hepatitis A and B immunization.
- Immunization against other diseases, e.g. yellow fever, may be needed if passing through another country.

Malaria is not a risk in Mecca (Makkah), Jeddah or Riyadh.

Hygiene

- Hand hygiene is vital.
- Many pilgrims wear face masks but benefits uncertain, especially as not all change them regularly.

Other

- Patients with diabetes or cardiovascular disease need special consideration.
- Sun protection may be needed, especially for men (who are more exposed).
- Travel insurance.
- Suitable footwear is needed for walking.

The practice nurse can help with some of these. There are also dedicated Hajj health clinics in the UK, as well as online resources. Farida is travelling in a family group and is already aware of many of the risks. She tells you she has already booked to attend a clinic in London for her jabs.

You ask her to return to see you in two months, after her pilgrimage, so you can check her BP and discuss whether she wants to continue on the Pill.

Resources

UK Medical Eligibility Criteria for Contraceptive Use (2009).
   http://www.fsrh.org/pdfs/UKMEC2009.pdf

Fit for Travel (from NHS Scotland).
   http://www.fitfortravel.nhs.uk/advice/general-travel-health-advice/hajj-and-umrah-pilgrimage.aspx

Health and travel advice for Hajj pilgrims (FCO, HM Government; updated annually).
   https://www.gov.uk/government/news/health-and-travel-advice-for-hajj-pilgrims

National Travel Health Network and Centre.
   http://www.nathnac.org/

CASE

40 It's my leg

Alan Jackson, age 67 years

Retired taxi driver

PMH: MI 2 yrs ago; mild COPD; back pain 10 years ago; shoulder injury

Medication: aspirin, amlodipine, simvastatin, Pulmicort and Bricanyl inhalers

---

Mr Jackson gestures towards his right knee and lower leg and says he's had pain 'for some time'. The foot can hurt at night too. It's a sort of burning pain. The leg 'gives out' when he walks, which is not far as a rule. You try to get more information about the pain and what makes it better or worse, but Mr Jackson doesn't give a very clear history. His other leg seems OK and he doesn't have pain anywhere else.

He retired from being a taxi driver nearly 10 years ago, following a shoulder injury. Two years ago he had a heart attack and he hasn't felt that well since. He doesn't have any hobbies really, just hangs around the house and gets 'under the missus's feet'. The doctors told him he should get regular exercise after his heart attack, but he never really got into it. He has been a smoker since his teens and drinks a 'moderate' amount of alcohol. There's no family history of diabetes. He's always been roughly the same weight, which is 93 kg. He is 1.66 m tall so his BMI is 33.7.

What are the possibilities at this stage? Write down five broad categories.

With this vague history, it could be one of several very different problems.
- **Musculoskeletal.** Here DJD of the knee and ankle are at the top of the list. Sciatica is also possible given his previous back trouble. It's unlikely to be gout, though gout can become chronic.
- **Neurogenic** pain, possibly diabetic neuropathy, neurogenic claudication from spinal stenosis, or an entrapment syndrome.
- **Peripheral vascular disease.** Intermittent claudication fits the history and is highly likely given his previous MI, obesity, smoking and sedentary lifestyle.
- **Deep vein thrombosis**.
- **Infection**, anything from cellulitis to osteomyelitis.
- **Tumour**. A primary tumour in the leg is unlikely in this age group, but it could be a secondary.
- Simple muscular **weakness** can cause legs to 'give out' but is unlikely to cause pain, especially unilateral.

You ask to examine him. His BP is 146/90 and pulse 82 regular. He rolls up his trouser leg and shows you a right shin which looks very pink, shiny and hairless. At this point you explain that you need to take a proper look at him.

What do you need to examine?

- **Both legs**, checking the state of the skin, the joints and the circulation, comparing both sides. Remember the femoral pulses too.

- **Spine** – check ROM and any tenderness.
- **Abdomen** – for aortic aneurysm.
- Consider examining the **chest**, including the heart for murmurs and other abnormalities.

Up on the couch, both lower legs now look pale. They are also hairless and slightly shiny, the right leg more so. The skin is intact, including over the feet, and you can feel femoral and popliteal pulses. Dorsalis pedis is absent on both sides, and posterior tibial absent on the right. His abdomen is obese but otherwise normal and his spine moves well.

What is the likely diagnosis?

Peripheral vascular disease with unilateral intermittent claudication. You also wonder if he sounds a bit depressed.

Peripheral vascular disease

About 10% of people have PVD, not always symptomatic. PVD increases with age.

Main risk factors
- other CV disease including ED
- smoking – the single most important modifiable risk factor
- DM
- hyperlipidaemia
- hypertension
- obesity
- hyperviscosity
- Buerger's disease
- Leriche syndrome.

High mortality rate: 50% at 5 years, 70% at 10 years.

Suspect chronic limb ischaemia if
- progressive-onset intermittent claudication
- unexplained foot pain at rest/at night
- absent or hard to feel peripheral pulses
- pallor on elevation and rubor on dependency (Buerger's sign)
- shiny hairless leg skin
- non-healing wounds on the lower limb.

Diagnosis is based on clinical features and ankle branchial pressure index (ABPI) <0.9 (normal >1).

Management
- reducing risk factors, especially smoking
- supervised exercise programme for intermittent claudication
- skin and foot care
- consider referral to vascular surgery unit.

Acute arterial occlusion can supervene or arise *de novo*. Can be caused by:
- plaque rupture or *in situ* thrombosis
- embolus from the heart or proximal arteries.

If there is already chronic limb ischaemia, collaterals may have developed.

General Practice Cases at a Glance, First Edition. Carol Cooper and Martin L Block. © 2017 John Wiley & Sons, Ltd. Published 2017 by John Wiley & Sons, Ltd.

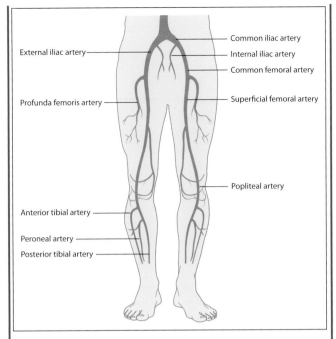

Figure 40.1 Arterial supply to the lower limb.

In theory, embolism is more serious for the leg than thrombosis as there may be collaterals in pre-existing PVD.

Always suspect arterial occlusion if there is:
- onset of leg pain over minutes, hours or days
- the '6 Ps' –

▶ pain
▶ pallor
▶ pulselessness
▶ paraesthesia
▶ paralysis
▶ perishing with cold.

If there are extensive collaterals, the leg may be dusky instead of pale.

Management
- Arrange immediate admission to vascular surgery.
- Revascularization (angioplasty or bypass surgery) may save the limb.
- Endartectomy is a good option for localized disease.

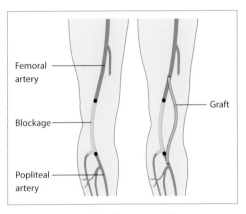

Figure 40.2 Femoro-popliteal bypass grafting.

You therefore tell Mr Jackson that it sounds like there's not enough blood going to the leg. This would account for his symptoms. You will try your best to help him. Does he consider he could stop smoking as this is very important?

He's not sure, and shrugs, adding, 'I might give it a go, if you say it's important'.

You arrange a blood test for FBC, CRP, U&E and creatinine, LFTs, lipids and HbA1c, and send him to the nurse for smoking cessation and hopefully weight loss in due course.

When you review him next week, consider:
- referral for vascular assessment
- changing his aspirin to clopidogrel
- lowering his cholesterol below 4.0 mmol/L
- exploring his mental state further.

If other measures fail to relieve his claudication, **naftidrofuryl** may help.

Mr Jackson returns in just 4 days. His leg pain is worse since the early hours of the morning.

Even before examining him, what are your thoughts?

You should be thinking of peripheral arterial occlusion due to thrombus or embolus. If you miss acute limb ischaemia, your patient could lose his limb and possibly his life. The family would also have a strong case against you.

You examine Mr Jackson and find that his right leg is pale and cool – almost cold, in fact. You cannot feel a popliteal pulse on the right.

What do you do now?

You should refer him immediately to the vascular surgery unit for admission.

What do you tell him?

It's probably best to keep it simple and tell him that his leg is really short of blood now, and a specialist should see him urgently, before things get too bad to treat, which can happen very quickly. Ask if he'd like you to speak to anyone, such as his wife.

Mr Jackson is admitted to hospital and has a femoro-popliteal bypass, with a stormy postoperative recovery due to his COPD.

Resources
CKS/NICE Peripheral arterial disease.
http://cks.nice.org.uk/peripheral-arterial-disease#!topicsummary
You might also like to try Case 4: 'My knee is very bad'.

CASE
41 I'm having terrible diarrhoea

John Baker, age 61 years
Betting shop manager
PMH: hypercholesterolaemia
Medication: atorvastatin 20 mg daily

Causes of acute diarrhoea

- Viruses, e.g. rotavirus, norovirus. This is the most common cause.
- Bacteria, e.g. *Campylobacter*, *Salmonella*, *Shigella*.
- Parasites, e.g. *Giardia*.
- Medications, e.g. metformin, antibiotics and many others (see BNF for more details).
- Acute anxiety.
- Acute serious bowel disease, such as:
  - appendicitis
  - ischaemic bowel.
- First presentation of chronic diarrhoea (see Causes box).

You have known Mr and Mrs Baker for several years. They both enjoy good health and see the GP infrequently. Mr Baker has booked in to see you in an emergency slot. You collect him from your waiting room, and he walks down the corridor looking a little tired and glum. He sits down, sighs, and you ask him what you can do for him today. Mr Baker tells you he is having 'terrible diarrhoea'.

What should your next question be?

You should start by asking an open question and giving Mr Baker time to talk. Patients will often speak uninterrupted for the first minute, and it is likely that during this time Mr Baker will give you the important information that you need. After this you can fill in the detail, first with more open questions then some specific closed questions.

A good open question here would be, 'Tell me more about the diarrhoea.'

Mr Baker tells you that he has been having diarrhoea for about five days now. He is rushing to the toilet about five times a day, and his stools are very watery. He felt a little sick at the beginning but this has now settled. He wonders if it might be caused by something he ate, but isn't really sure what this might be. His wife has been well. They often babysit for their granddaughter Bethany who is two years old. It's not uncommon for her to bring home illnesses, but this time she seems fine.

Through asking an open question and listening, you have lots of useful information about this current illness and on Mr Baker's perspective about what he thinks going on. Mr Baker is presenting you the facts he thinks you need to know. Now it is time for you to fill in the gaps.

What else should you be exploring in your consultation?

Find out **more about the current illness**. You are already clear about duration and frequency. Now you should ask specifically about:
- presence of **blood**
- **fever**
- **pain**.

Explore the **possible causes**. You should cover:
- any contact history
- any recent travel
- any new medications
- any recent stress.

Assess the level of **dehydration**.
- How is the urine output?
- How is the fluid intake?
- Are there any other symptoms such as light-headedness and weakness?

Mr Baker confirms there are no other symptoms. There is no blood, no fever and no significant pain. He can't think of anyone he knows who has had diarrhoea recently. He laughs when you ask him about recent travel, referring to a recent long weekend with his wife to Margate. He's been doing his best to keep drinking plenty of fluids, but in spite of this he reckons he is probably passing less urine than normal, and it seems more concentrated than usual.

What examination should you do?

You should check Mr Baker's basic observations and examine his abdomen. Consider doing a PR examination.

You find his pulse is 84 and regular, BP 139/86 and temperature 36.7 °C. His abdomen is soft and a little bloated. There is no significant tenderness. Bowel sounds are present.

What is the most likely cause?

It is most likely that Mr Baker has a viral illness. The absence of other symptoms, such as blood, pain or fever, go against this being a bacterial illness. The presence of these symptoms would make you want to check a stool sample.

Is Mr Baker dehydrated?

Mr Baker's decrease in urine output and increasingly concentrated urine suggest a mild/moderate level of dehydration. His normal pulse and BP suggest this is not severe.

How would you explain your diagnosis?

Your explanation should be clear and concise. Something like, 'Mr Baker, the most likely cause for your diarrhoea is that you have a virus. This is an illness that you have probably caught from somebody and is causing your bowel to become very sensitive. The virus should not last too long before the body clears it. In the meantime, the most important thing is to drink enough fluid to prevent you getting dehydrated.'

What advice should you offer?

Stress the importance of hydration. Mr Baker may find simple oral rehydration like Dioralyte helpful. Were Mr Baker showing evidence of severe diarrhoea you would consider admission.

General Practice Cases at a Glance, First Edition. Carol Cooper and Martin L Block. © 2017 John Wiley & Sons, Ltd. Published 2017 by John Wiley & Sons, Ltd.

It is also important to have a clear safety net, outlining when further follow-up would be needed.

What should you cover in your safety net?

There are two important areas here.

Deterioration in the current illness:
- increasing levels of pain or fever
- signs of dehydration (e.g. further reduction in urine output).

Persistence of symptoms to suggest a chronic condition:
- symptoms persisting at four weeks of illness.

Mr Baker thanks you for your clear explanation and helpful advice and leaves.

Next month Mr Baker returns to see you as he remembers you advising him to come back if his diarrhoea did not get better after a month. He tells you that it has been six weeks now. Although things are slightly better than before (he is only going three times a day), and there are no other new symptoms like blood or fever, he decided it was worth coming back.

What needs to happen now?

Mr Baker now satisfies the suspected lower GI cancer guidance for referral under the two-week pathway.

Suspected lower GI cancer guidelines

Refer under the two-week rule if:
- 40+ with rectal bleeding with a change of bowel habit towards looser stools and/or increased stool frequency persisting for six weeks
- 60+ with rectal bleeding persisting for six weeks or more without a change in bowel habit and without anal symptoms, an urgent referral should be made
- 60+ with a change in bowel habit to looser stools and/or more frequent stools persisting for six weeks or more without rectal bleeding

---

- right lower abdominal mass or palpable rectal mass
- men of any age with unexplained iron-deficiency anaemia and a haemoglobin of 11 g/100 mL
- non-menstruating women with unexplained iron-deficiency anaemia and a haemoglobin of 10 g/100 mL or below.

You explain to Mr Baker that because of the persisting symptoms of diarrhoea he needs to be seen in an urgent clinic where he will see specialist doctors who will do tests to exclude cancer. Mr Baker looks a little shocked but is happy that his ongoing symptoms are being taken seriously.

Three weeks later you receive a letter from clinic. Mr Baker has had a normal colonoscopy and has been given a diagnosis of post-infectious irritable bowel syndrome.

Causes of chronic diarrhoea

- Irritable bowel syndrome.
- Chronic infection.
- Inflammatory bowel disease (e.g. ulcerative colitis or Crohn's disease).
- Coeliac disease.
- Microscopic colitis.
- Diverticular disease.
- Colon cancer.

Resources

Nice cancer guidance.
 https://www.nice.org.uk/guidance/cg27/
CKS/NICE Gastroenteritis.
 http://cks.nice.org.uk/gastroenteritis
BNF.org

You may also like to try Case 12: 'My baby has an upset tummy' and Case 10: 'It's my back passage'.

CASE 42

The nurse did my diabetes check last week. I'm here for the results

Sahra Ali, age 59 years
Unemployed
PMH: type 2 diabetes; hypertension; no complications
Medication: metformin 1 g tds, atorvastatin 40 mg od, ramipril 10 mg od

Mrs Ali and her family are longstanding patients at your practice. The family are from Somalia and are Muslim. You see from your system that Mrs Ali is seeing you for follow-up after her annual diabetic review with the practice nurse. According to the nurse review:

- urine dipstick clear
- BP 127/74
- no evidence of peripheral neuropathy
- non-smoker
- recent diabetic eye check – no evidence of eye disease
- BMI – 29 (up from 26 last year).

Her blood and urine results are also available (Table 42.1).

Mrs Ali comes in to your room and sits down. She is keen to know what her blood results are.

What is the important result here?

Mrs Ali's Hba1c has deteriorated since her last review. This is in the context of her BMI increasing too.

How should you address this in the consultation?

You should first explain the results to Mrs Ali, specifically that her Hba1c reading (which is an indicator of an average blood sugar over the last three months) has got worse since last year. You need to be sure that Mrs Ali understands what this means and the importance of controlling this well, to decrease the risk of future complications. Find out if she knows what these might be. If not, give a brief outline (e.g. 'heart disease, kidney trouble and eye problems that can't be fixed with glasses').

Ensure you bring Mrs Ali into this discussion. Does she understand her condition? Does she have friends or relatives with diabetes? Does she have a target reading and importantly **does she have any idea why her sugars have gone up this last year**?

Mrs Ali tells you that she is not that surprised that her sugar level has gone up. She has had a bad year. Her mother died a few months ago, and her eldest daughter's marriage broke down in the summer and she moved back into the family home. She is

feeling less down about things now, but she knows she had a period of overeating, especially sweet puddings and cakes. This is more under control now, but she did put on weight and this probably made matters worse.

> **Tip**
>
> **Don't assume the patient understands the condition.** In chronic disease management the initial consultations are vital in helping a patient understand their condition and the rationale behind the treatment. However, you can never assume the level of understanding in future review appointments. It is worth checking this and if necessary going back to a conversation about the diagnosis.
>
> The **Diabetes UK** website is a good resource here. You can also refer back to a diabetes education course such as the **DESMOND** course.

What should you aim to achieve in the consultation today?

By the end of this consultation you and Mrs Ali should have agreed on a plan to bring the sugars down. It is really important that Mrs Ali has ownership of this plan, and that it fits into her life.

What are your options? Name two.

- Bring the Hba1c down with **diet** and **exercise.**
- Bring the Hba1c down with further **medical treatment** (e.g. gliclazide or insulin).

You outline the above with Mrs Ali. She is really keen to do all she can to bring the Hba1c down through improving her diet and exercise. She has recently joined a local walking group, but she isn't sure about what she can do to improve her diet.

> **Principals of healthy eating in type 2 diabetes**
>
> **Fruit and vegetables**
> Aim for five a day – mix of colours.
>
> **Carbohydrate**
> - Choose slowly absorbed (low GI) carbohydrate – ideally wholemeal.
> - Limit portion size.
> - Spread throughout the day.
>
> **Sugars**
> - Try to limit as much as possible.
> - Avoid any sugars in drinks (including fruit juice).
>
> **Fats**
> Try to limit as much as possible.
>
> **Protein, e.g. meat, fish, pulses**
> Include some food from this group every day.
>
> **Salt**
> Limit to <6 g/day

Table 42.1 Mrs Ali's test results.

	Last year	This year
Hba1c	51 mmol/mol (6.8%)	65 mmol/mol (8.1%)
Cholesterol	3.4 mmol/L	3.8 mmol/L
U+E	Normal	Normal

What could you do to help her with this?

You have a few options at your fingertips.

- Refer her back to a diabetes **education course** (e.g. DESMOND).
- Signpost her to some useful resources (such as the **Diabetes UK** website, which has a useful section on recipes, lots of clear patient information and advice. The section on managing diabetes during Ramadan may be useful for Mrs Ali.)
- Refer her to the **practice nurse** or a **dietician** to discuss further.

What is the DESMOND programme?

The DESMOND programme is a diabetes education course run in the community for people with or at risk of type 2 diabetes. It is delivered by trained healthcare professionals and lay educators and covers useful information and practical ways to manage (or prevent) type 2 diabetes. It is recommended that all newly diagnosed type 2 diabetics attend this course, but it is also available to those with longstanding type 2 diabetes who nee a 'top-up'. There is a similar course for type 1 diabetics (DAPHNE).

You show Mrs Ali the recipe section on the Diabetes UK website which she reads with interest. She is also keen to go back to the DESMOND course. It is a while since she last attended, she is keen to go back and learn some more.

You close the consultation by asking Mrs Ali what her targets are. She is clear that she wants to bring her sugars and weight down through a mix of healthy diet and exercise. She has a plan that she intends to stick to. She wants to stay healthy for as long as possible! She tells you that she will see you in a few months time and you will see the difference.

Six months later Mrs Ali books in to see you again having had a repeat Hba1c blood test.

- Her new Hba1c level is 52 mmol/mol (6.9%).
- Her BMI is also back down to 26.

She is over the moon to have brought this back down naturally, and she is grateful to you for helping to do this.

Resources

Diabetes UK.
  https://www.diabetes.org.uk
CKS/NICE Type 2 diabetes.
  http://cks.nice.org.uk/diabetes-type-2

43 My skin is really itchy

Chloe Chen, age 8 years
PMH: nil of note
Medication: nil

Chloe is booked in to see you today. You've seen her twice before and she seems to recognize you. You confirm that the person bringing her in today is (as you suspected) her mum. She introduces herself as Sao Chen. Chloe sits down next to mum and you ask Chloe what you can do for her. Chloe goes on to say, 'My skin is really itchy. Especially at night. Sometimes I itch all night.' At this point mum chips in with, 'We tried using some Sudocrem and some E45, and neither makes it any better.'

What questions do you want to ask now? Think of at least four.

- 'Is there any rash? If so, where?'
- 'How long has it been going on for?'
- 'Have you noticed any **triggers**?' There may be pets, stress or changes in diet.
- 'Is this something Chloe has had before?'
- 'Does anyone in the **family** have eczema, asthma or hay fever?'
- 'Is there any **pain**?' Its presence suggests bacterial infection.
- 'How long has the mother tried the treatments for?'

Chloe and her mum go on to say that the itching is worse inside both of her elbows and on her hands. She has had some itching

before on her face but this is fine now. They haven't noticed any triggers, though they have just had some building work done at home, and this made the place very dusty. Things have been worse over the last month. It is not sore. Mrs Chen has tried Sudocrem for a couple of weeks to no avail. She started using E45 over the week-end, which does not seem to have helped much either. Mum goes on to say that she had eczema as a child, but that she grew out of it.

Describe your examination

Firstly you should tell Chloe and her mum what you would like to do. You are **signposting** the upcoming examination.

Your examination should include observation of any itchy areas of skin, and a **general** assessment of the skin.

You examine Chloe, and you find that she has dry excoriated skin on both antecubital fossae and on both of her hands (notably on her second, third and fourth fingers and the anterior surface of her hands bilaterally). This is a little red in places. The rest of her skin seems largely normal.

What is your diagnosis?

Chloe has a likely diagnosis of atopic eczema.

How would you describe this diagnosis?

Try to explain the diagnosis to both mother and child in as **child-friendly** language as possible. Something like, 'You have eczema, which means your skin can feel dry and itchy. Sometimes this gets worse because something sets it off (like dust or pets). There are

Table 43.1 Common itchy skin rashes in children.

Condition	Details
Atopic eczema	Dry excoriated skin Bilateral typically May be exacerbated by triggers Treat as described in text
Ringworm	Well demarcated round lesion(s) Unilateral Treat with antifungal cream
Scabies	Widespread intense itching and excoriation Rash all over body Mite burrows in between fingers Topical treatments (such as permethrin cream)

General Practice Cases at a Glance, First Edition. Carol Cooper and Martin L Block. © 2017 John Wiley & Sons, Ltd. Published 2017 by John Wiley & Sons, Ltd.

lots of things you can do and we can help make things get better.' This should be backed up with a patient information leaflet (e.g. from patient.co.uk). You should check with Chloe and her mum that they understand what is going on.

> **Tip**
>
> **Pain in eczema = infection.**
> New onset of pain in the presence of atopic eczema is likely to represent bacterial infection. This should be treated with a course of oral antibiotics (e.g. oral flucloxacillin for one week).

Chloe and her mum both nod, and the mum asks, 'Will she grow out of it?'

Will Chloe grow out of it?

Her mother grew out of it, and many children do, so there is a good chance that she will grow out of it. You can say that hopefully she will, but that you cannot know for sure.

What are the main themes you should discuss in your management plan?

- Emollient usage.
- Conservative measures (such as **trigger avoidance**).
- Short-term courses of **topical steroid** cream.
- Anti-itching medication (e.g. **antihistamine** at night).

It may be worth exploring if mum is thinking about using any herbal treatments and discouraging this when it is inappropriate.

Describe how she should use her emollients

Regularly. In eczema the skin's ability to maintain hydration breaks down and this worsens the condition. Regular emollient is essential and must be kept up. Sudocrem is not an effective emollient (it is a barrier cream used commonly to prevent or treat nappy rash). She has tried E45, but maybe not for long enough.

What conservative measures could she try?

You should recommend simple measures as shown here.

> **Conservative measures in atopic eczema**
>
> - Avoid scratching the eczema.
> - Keep the nails short.
> - Avoid trigger factors.

This will also be described in most patient information leaflets. Along with antihistamine medication, this will be helpful in breaking the itch–scratch cycle.

How should she tackle potential triggers?

Chloe and her family should try to identify any possible triggers though their own observation, and try avoiding potential common triggers.

> **Common triggers in atopic eczema**
>
> - Food, e.g. milk, egg, wheat, soy, peanut.
> - Irritants, e.g. soap, detergent.
> - Heat, particularly hand washing with hot water.
> - Fabrics, e.g. synthetic fabrics and wool.
> - Inhaled allergens, e.g. house dust mite, pollen.
> - Stress.
> - Hormonal.

Should you use steroid cream?

It is possible that, with regular emollient and appropriate conservative measures, Chloe's eczema will settle without the need for topical steroids. However if it doesn't, or it gets worse, then she may benefit from topical steroids. The strength of the steroid cream or ointment used should relate to the severity of the flare-up, and should ideally be used for the shortest period possible, stopping 2 days after the flare-up has settled.

> **Steroid creams**
>
> - Mild: hydrocortisone 1% (can be used on the face).
> - Moderate: Eumovate.
> - Potent: Betnovate.
> - Very potent: Dermovate.

Chloe's mum decides that they would like to avoid steroid cream in the first instance, but will come back to see you if things aren't getting better. You prescribe an emollient ointment to use both during the flare-up (in large quantities) and regularly (in lesser quantities) afterwards.

Chloe and her mum leave with your prescription and an information leaflet, hopeful of some improvement.

Resources

CKS/NICE Eczema.
   http://cks.nice.org.uk/eczema-atopic
Patient information.
   http://www.patient.co.uk/health/atopic-eczema

Doctor, I'm just feeling really down

> **James McCormack, age 54 years**
> Fork-lift truck driver
> PMH: type 2 diabetes
> Medication: metformin 500 mg bd, ramipril 5 mg od, simvastatin 40 mg nocte

Mr McCormack sits down with a weary look and says quietly, 'Doctor, I'm just feeling really down at the moment. Is there anything you can do to help me?' At this point he starts crying and you offer him a tissue.

What would you do next?

This is probably a moment where you should step back. If you go in too quickly with lots of questions you might close down the consultation. Step back, allow him a little space, and listen.

With you offering not much more than a look of warmth and sympathy Mr McCormack continues with his story.

'Doctor, things have got really bad. I'm never normally like this, but, I don't know, it's just I'm really, really down. I lost my job at the end of last year. After almost 20 years with the firm. I haven't been able to find work since and now we're really struggling. Things have gone downhill since then. I can't sleep, I can't eat, I'm barely leaving the house. I sit there just crying most nights. I can hardly even watch the TV, it's that bad. My wife doesn't know what to do with me. She pushed me to come here today. It's really bad, really bad, doc.'

What would you do now?

Again, don't rush in with more questions just yet. It's probably a good moment to offer some words of humanity such as, 'I'm sorry to hear this'. At which point Mr McCormack says, 'Thank you, doctor. I've never felt like this before.'

What questions would you need to ask to explore the depression further?

There are some key areas you need to cover here.

Firstly, **understanding** and **exploring** his depression. Mr McCormack has given you lots of information already, but it may be useful to clarify some areas.

- 'Have you been getting any **pleasure** out of doing things?'
- 'Tell me more about your **sleeping**.'
- 'How is your **concentration**?'
- 'Are you drinking **alcohol** at the moment?'

Mr McCormack confirms he is getting hardly any pleasure from life. He used to enjoy fishing, but hasn't done this for ages. The only thing that makes him smile is when he gets to see his grandchildren. His daughter brings them over a couple of times a week.

They are 18 months and four years of age. His sleep is poor most nights, often waking up at 4am. He's not really drinking much alcohol at the moment. He used to go down the pub at the weekend, but hasn't felt like doing this recently.

Secondly, understanding the **impact** that depression is having on Mr McCormack. Try asking, 'How has this been affecting you?'

Mr McCormack explains how his depression is affecting his relationship with his wife and is making it difficult for him to motivate himself to try and find work.

Importantly you need to **assess suicide risk**. Suicidal thoughts are common in depression, and patients are often reassured to know that this is the case.

What questions would you ask here to assess his risk of suicide?

Useful questions include:
- 'Have you been feeling like harming yourself?'
- 'Have you had any thought of suicide?'
- 'Have you made any plans?'
- 'Do you have the means for doing this?'
- 'What has kept you from acting on these thoughts?'

Mr McCormack wells up again when you ask him about this. He has had thoughts of suicide, but knows he wouldn't act on them. The thought of his little grandchildren keeps him from wanting to act on them.

What is the diagnosis here?

Mr McCormack has severe depression.

What are your management options?

In moderate to severe depression patients should be offered:
- **antidepressants** (SSRIs are the first-line option)
- **psychological** therapy.

It is also worth exploring lifestyle factors such as:
- **exercise** and generally being active
- **social activity**, seeing friends and family
- offering advice about **sleep** hygiene.

Finally, it is worth asking patients with depression, 'What do you think you could do that would make the biggest difference?' Often people have a good idea of what might help.

When would you follow up Mr McCormack?

It would be reasonable to review Mr McCormack in 2–3 weeks. It will take this long for the SSRI to start to work. He should be offered the option of returning sooner if things get worse.

Resources
CKS/NICE Depression.
http://cks.nice.org.uk/depression
You may also like to try Case 37: 'I'm all over the place these days'.

I've got a really bad burning in my stomach

Mrs Halima Akhber, age 39 years
Housewife
PMH: nil of note
Medication: nil at present

Mrs Halima Akhber comes to see you. She has come in today as over the past couple of months she has been troubled by 'a really bad burning in the stomach'. It makes her feel sick. It gets worse when she eats. She has tried some Gaviscon from the pharmacist. This helped a bit, but did not get rid of the pain. She works as a nursery nurse and is now getting fed up as she has had to miss a couple of days from work last week because of the pain.

As you listen further she tells you that her grandfather died of cancer of the stomach last year and she is worried that this might be what is happening to her.

As you have given Halima time to talk she has given you lots of useful information about her problem, how it is affecting her, and what is in the back of her mind (her grandfather's cancer).

What are your initial thoughts on the likely diagnosis? Write down three possibilities.

- Dyspepsia.
- Peptic ulcer.
- IBS.
- Malignancy (less likely but you need to exclude any alarm features).

Red flags to suggest malignancy – require urgent referral

- ► Chronic gastrointestinal bleeding.
- ► Progressive unintentional weight loss.
- ► Progressive difficulty swallowing.
- ► Persistent vomiting.
- ► Iron-deficiency anaemia.
- ► Epigastric mass.
- ► People over 55 years of age with persistent or unexplained recent-onset dyspepsia.

What questions might help you exclude red flags?

- 'Has there been any weight loss?'
- 'Have you had any problems swallowing?'
- 'Any vomiting?'
- 'Any blood when you open your bowels?'
Fortunately her answers are all negative.

Are there any medications you should enquire about?

Yes. It's always worth asking about **NSAIDs** (non-steroidal anti-inflammatory drugs, e.g. ibuprofen) which she may be buying over the counter.

Mrs Akhber tells you she hasn't taken any other medication apart from the Gaviscon.

What about lifestyle factors? Any of these you should enquire about?

Yes. Smoking and alcohol can both aggravate acid dyspepsia. In this case Mrs Akhber neither smokes nor drinks alcohol.

It may be worth checking if she has noticed if any food or drink makes an impact. Again in this case there is nothing specific, but she does say that it can be worse when she gets really hungry.

Lifestyle factors that may worsen dyspepsia

- Obesity.
- Smoking.
- Alcohol intake.
- Stress.
- Going to bed on a full stomach.

What key questions will your examination help you to answer?

Your examination now should help you:
- clarify your diagnosis
- confirm absence of an acute abdomen or GI bleeding that would require admission
- confirm absence of signs of malignancy.

On examination:
- her pulse is 74
- her weight is 94 kg, giving her a BMI of 31.4
- her abdomen is soft, there is mild tenderness in the epigastrium but no palpable mass
- there is no guarding to suggest peritonism.

What is your working diagnosis?

The history and examination suggest a diagnosis of acid dyspepsia. There are no alarm features to suggest malignancy.

How would you explain this diagnosis in clear language the patient understands?

Try what works for you. A good example may be 'Your stomach has become sore because of the stomach acid burning the lining.'

It may be worth specifically addressing the issue of malignancy by stating that there are no features from her history or her examination to suggest cancer.

What are your management options?

- Lifestyle: Mrs Akhber would benefit from **losing some weight**. She may also want to look at the type of food that aggravates her symptoms, a food diary may be useful here.
- Testing for ***Helicobacter pylori***.
- Treatment with a **PPI**: you should give one month of full-dose PPI (e.g. omeprazole 20 mg). If this has not settled the symptoms then you should review Mrs Akhber at the end of the treatment.

Resources

CKS/NICE Dyspepsia.
http://cks.nice.org.uk/dyspepsia-unidentified-cause

I want to talk about my risk of breast cancer

Desta Gebru, age 36 years
Accountant
PMH: mild asthma
Medication: salbutamol 100 µg inhaler 2 puffs qds prn

Ms Gebru is a newly registered patient at your practice. She was born in Ethiopia but has lived in the UK for the last 16 years. She is booked into a routine slot in your Tuesday afternoon clinic. She sits down and says, 'I want to talk about my risk of breast cancer.' You ask her to tell you more and she continues. 'My sister and I were both talking about how there has been a lot of women in our family with cancer. Lots of breast cancer. I decided it was important that I get checked out.'

What do you need to do now in your history?

You need to map out a **family tree** for Ms Gebru to include:
• any cancer cases (not just breast) in all known relatives (up to third degree – see Table 46.1), both female and male cases
• any known faulty genes (BRCA1, BRCA2, TP53)
• age at onset
• bilateral or unilateral
• any Ashkenazi Jewish ancestry.

You sit down with Ms Gebru and talk through her family history. She is the youngest of seven children, four of whom are girls.
• Her oldest sister Senalat was diagnosed with unilateral breast cancer at the age of 43. She died a year later.
• Her mother is well and is one of three sisters.
• Her aunt Zena (mother's older sister) died of breast cancer. This was a long time ago and she does not remember much more about it.

Her aunt Fana (mother's middle sister) died of ovarian cancer she does not have any more details.

All these family members were diagnosed and treated back in Ethiopia. She is not aware of the results of any genetic testing.

There is no additional history that she is aware of in her family. Both her grandparents died of natural causes and there is no cancer on her father's side of the family, and no history of male cancers that she is aware of.

Have a go at drawing a family tree for Ms Gebru

You draw a simple family tree, and share this with Ms Gebru for confirmation (Figure 46.1).

Table 46.1 Degrees of relatives.

Degree of relative	Relative
First degree	Mother, father, daughter, son, sister, brother
Second degree	Grandparents, grandchildren, aunt, uncle, niece, nephew, half-sister, half-brother
Third degree	Great-grandparents, great-grandchildren, great-aunt, great-uncle, first cousin, grand-nephew, grand-niece

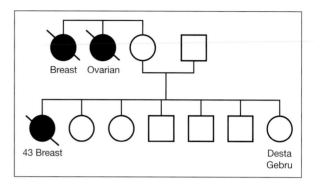

Figure 46.1 Family tree for Desta Gebru.

What else should you ask Ms Gebru in your history?

• Has she noticed any changes in her breast?
• Has she ever had any children and, if so, did she breastfeed?

Ms Gebru confirms that she has not noticed any changes to her breast, and she has never had any children.

Should Ms Gebru be referred to the breast cancer family history clinic?

Yes, she should be referred. She has one first-degree and one second-degree relative with breast cancer, and one second-degree relative diagnosed with ovarian cancer. Regardless of their age of onset she warrants onwards referral.

Criteria for referral to secondary care

• One first-degree female relative diagnosed with breast cancer under the age of 40 years.
• One first-degree male relative diagnosed with breast cancer at any age.
• One first-degree relative with bilateral breast cancer where the first primary was diagnosed under the age of 50 years.
• Two first-degree relatives, or one first-degree and one second-degree relative, diagnosed with breast cancer at any age.
• One first-degree or second-degree relative diagnosed with breast cancer at any age and one first-degree or second-degree relative diagnosed with ovarian cancer at any age (one of these should be a first-degree relative).
• Three first-degree or second-degree relatives diagnosed with breast cancer at any age.
From cks.nice.org.uk/breast-cancer-managing-fh

What should you say to Ms Gebru about next steps?

You should give a clear, jargon-free explanation about the next steps, that is that you are referring her to a family history clinic where it is likely she will be offered genetic testing. Try something like, 'Because of the family history you have shared with me, there is a chance that you might have a gene that increases your chance of developing breast cancer. I'd like to refer you to a family history clinic. They will see you, ask some more questions and offer you some tests to screen for these faulty genes.' This explanation has given Ms Gebru an indication of what to expect in the next steps.

General Practice Cases at a Glance, First Edition. Carol Cooper and Martin L Block. © 2017 John Wiley & Sons, Ltd. Published 2017 by John Wiley & Sons, Ltd.

You explain this to Ms Gebru who takes it in stoically. She was expecting this would be the case and she is grateful that she is being taken seriously.

Ms Gebru attends the breast cancer family history clinic at your local hospital. She is counselled further and opts to undertake genetic screening for breast cancer. She is aware that if one of the genetic tests is positive she may be offered mastectomy.

The follow-up letter from clinic informs you that Ms Gebru was tested for the presence of recognised genes linked to breast cancer and that all these were normal. The advice from clinic is that Ms Gebru follow the simple measures (outlined in the box) to monitor her breasts and to decrease her risk of future breast cancer.

You see Ms Gebru in clinic the following month to discuss her appointment. She was a little unclear about the advice and she wanted to check this with you. She is relieved she does not have any of these faulty genes and she will do her best to decrease her risk in the future.

Women at increased risk of breast cancer

- Should all be **'breast aware'**.
- Should be familiar with what is normal and report changes (e.g. discomfort, pain, lumps, thickening, nipple changes or discharge and skin changes).

The following can **reduce the risk of breast cancer**:
- physical exercise
- maintenance of a healthy weight
- reduction of alcohol intake
- having a first child at a younger age
- breastfeeding.

Ms Gebru tells you that she will be increasing her level of exercise. She tells you how relieved she is to not have one of the 'breast cancer genes'. She is due to be married in the summer and is keen to start a family. She does not want her children to lose their mother to cancer like her cousins did.

All women in the UK are entitled to screening through the **NHS Breast Screening Programme** as outlined in the box.

NHS Breast Screening Programme

- Offered to all women aged 50–70 years every three years
- Currently being extended throughout England to include women aged 47–73 years.
- Women who are older than the maximum eligible screening age in their area can self-refer.

Resources

National Institute for Health and Care Excellence (NICE) Familial breast cancer: classification and care of people at risk of familial breast cancer and management of breast cancer and related risks in people with a family history of breast cancer (NICE, 2013).

NHS Breast Screening Programme.
http://www.cancerscreening.nhs.uk/breastscreen/

Cancer Research UK.
http://www.cancerresearchuk.org/about-cancer/cancers-in-general/causes-symptoms/genes-and-inherited-cancer-risk/

CASE
47
I've got a terrible back ache

Ray Watkins, age 54 years

Carpenter

PMH: kidney stones

Medication: nil

Mr Watkins has booked into an emergency slot in your Wednesday morning surgery. He was last seen in the practice just over six years ago, with a bout of flu, and, looking back through his notes, he is not a man to trouble the doctor. You go to the waiting room and call Mr Watkins. He stands up slowly, wincing as he hobbles down the corridor to your consulting room.

You ask Mr Watkins what you can do for him. He shakes his head and says 'I've got this terrible back ache, doctor.' You ask him to tell you more and he continues. 'It started about three weeks ago, I was stretching at work and I felt a twinge. It wasn't so bad straight away but it got worse overnight. I was laid up for about a week in bed. I tried to go in last week but I was in too much pain and I saw another doctor who signed me off for a couple of weeks. To be honest things aren't getting any better and there's no way I'm fit to go back as things stand.'

What do you think the patient wants out of the consultation today?

- He wants some relief for his back pain.
- He may also want a doctor's note for work.

What else would you like to find out about the back pain?

You should ask the following questions.
- Where is the pain?
- Does it move to anywhere?
- Any symptoms into your **legs** (such as pain, loss of power or sensation)?
- Any **bladder** or **bowel** symptoms?
- When is the pain worse?
- Any rest pain or night pain?
- Any **fever**?
- What have you tried taking for the pain?

Mr Watkins tells you that the main focus of the pain is the low back. There is some radiation into the right gluteal region, but no pain or weakness in his legs. The pain is worse when he tries to do things, and improves when he lies flat in bed. He's been trying to lie still as much as possible as he hopes this will improve matters. There is less pain at night, and there are no bladder or bowel symptoms and no fever. He tried some ibuprofen given to him by the previous GP for a couple of days, but this didn't seem to help.

What type of back pain do you think Mr Watkins has?

From what you know at this point it is likely that this is mechanical back pain, brought on by a minor strain three weeks ago.

How would you find out about the impact this is having on Mr Watkins' life?

An open question would be good here. Try something like, 'Tell me more about the effect this back pain is having on your life.'

You ask Mr Watkins this question and he replies, 'A terrible impact. I can't get back to work, I'm no use round the home and my wife is getting fed up with this situation.'

Describe your examination

You should begin by **exposing the back** fully. Take a good look for any deformity. **Palpate** the back area to feel for deformity or any areas of pain. Assess **movements** by asking him to bend forward and move his back to either side.

Ask him to lie on the couch and assess his lower limbs for neurological signs, specifically:
- any signs of weakness
- any loss of sensation
- any change in tone
- any loss or asymmetry of reflexes.

Perform a 'straight leg raise' to assess for nerve root pain (sciatica). This examination involves the patient lying on their back, while you lift each straight leg upwards in turn. Nerve root pain is often precipitated by this movement, with a shooting pain occurring down the leg at a specific degree of upward raise.

Mr Watkins' examination reveals a diffusely uncomfortable low back, but with no focal areas of deformity. Movement in all directions is restricted by pain and stiffness. There are no positive neurological signs of the lower limbs and both straight raises demonstrate no signs of sciatica.

Red flags in low back pain assessment

► Bladder dysfunction or faecal incontinence (? cauda equina syndrome).
► Rest pain or night pain (? malignancy, ? inflammatory arthritis).
► Sweats, weight loss (? malignancy, ? infection).
► Severe progressive neurological deficit (? cauda equina syndrome).
► Saddle anaesthesia – around perianal region (? cauda equina syndrome).

Now what type of back pain do you think Mr Watkins has?

It is very likely that your initial suspicions are correct, and that Mr Watkins does have mechanical low back pain.

Back pain

Mechanical (or non-specific) back pain. 95%+ of cases
- Absence of significant neurological features (history or examination).
- Initially following strain or injury and aggravated by movement.
- Absence of red flags.
- Improves with analgesia.
Treat with analgesia, mobilize +/– physiotherapy.

Nerve root pain (often called sciatica). <5% of cases
- Pain is associated with neurological features (history or examination).
- Pain may be severe and continue at rest.

May need further imaging and assessment. First-line treatment often analgesia and physiotherapy.

Cauda equina syndrome – rare
- Pressure on nerves of lower spinal cord.
- Low back pain and ► associated leg weakness, ► saddle anaesthesia and ► bladder dysfunction or ► faecal incontinence.
- ► Severe progressive neurological deficit.

Medical emergency.

Osteoarthritis

Common cause of chronic low back pain. Can have acute mechanical flare-ups which are treated as above.

Inflammatory arthritis

(e.g. ankylosing spondylitis)
- Chronic low back pain.
- Younger patients.
- Tender spine on examination.
- Morning stiffness.
- Often worse with rest.

Malignancy

(e.g. myeloma or metastatic disease)
- Ongoing pain.
- Night pain/rest pain.
- Other associated symptoms (e.g. sweats, weight loss).

Infection

(e.g. osteomyelitis)
- ► On-going atypical pain.
- ► Fever.

You confirm with Mr Watkins that you think his low back pain is mechanical in nature and was brought on by a minor strain at work.

What are the principles of your management?

- Analgesia.
- Mobilization.
- Return to normal activities as soon as possible.
- Physiotherapy if not settling.

You outline these above principles to Mr Watkins. He is a little surprised as he always thought that 'you should lie as still as possible with backache'. He is keen to return to work as soon as he can, but he tells you that he would really struggle as his work is very physical. He would be keen to try some alternative analgesia and is keen to consider physiotherapy, 'anything that will make the pain go away'.

You discuss analgesia. What is your guide?

You should use the analgesic ladder (see box). You should advise regular use of analgesia in the acute phase to keep on top of the pain.

The analgesic ladder

Step one
Paracetamol 1 g qds

Step two
Add in non-steroidal anti-inflammatory (NSAID). Ibuprofen 400 mg tds is standard, naproxen 500 mg bd is stronger.

Step three
Add in opiate, e.g. codeine phosphate 15 mg qds prn.
Step up by increasing strength of opiate.
Beware: addictive potential.

You prescribe regular paracetamol and naproxen (with PPI cover for the NSAID, omeprazole 20 mg od). You also make an urgent physiotherapy referral, marking on the form that Mr Watkins is currently unable to work due to his back pain.

Mr Watkins asks you to sign him off for three months to give him time to get better.

What should your approach to Mr Watkins' fit note be?

You should aim to sign Mr Watkins off for short periods of time with regular review. Long-term outcomes are worse the longer the individual is signed off for initially, with longer initial periods of being signed of work being associated with long-term sickness. Your aim should be to get him to a position of being able to return to work as soon as possible. Encourage him to mobilize and resume normal activities as much as possible. You sign Mr Watkins off for two weeks and arrange a review appointment.

In two weeks you see Mr Watkins, he has just started physiotherapy and is showing some signs of progress. He is hopeful he might be well enough to go back in two further weeks' time and you agree this period for your next fit note. This is indeed the case. Mr Watkins returns to work at this point, subsequently completing his course of physiotherapy and achieving a full recovery.

Resources

CKS/NICE Back pain – low (without radiculopathy).
   http://cks.nice.org.uk/back-pain-low-without-radiculopathy
CKS/NICE Sciatica (lumbar radiculopathy).
   http://cks.nice.org.uk/sciatica-lumbar-radiculopathy

CASE

48 I'd like antibiotics please

Sanjiv Patel, age 25 years
Works in retail
PMH: acne; meniscus injury
Medication: nil

Sanjiv rarely attends the surgery but today he has a sore throat which started just two days ago. It hurts to swallow and he had a little earache last night. Although he feels OK, he is asking for antibiotics.

He is a non-smoker and occasional drinker. He lives with his parents and his two sisters. There has been no recent travel.

How do you respond to his request for antibiotics?

If you tell him now that antibiotics won't help, you risk alienating him. While it is true that most sore throats are viral and self-limiting, you do not yet have enough information to know whether Sanjiv would benefit from an antibiotic.

Sore throat

- Can be due to adenovirus, parainfluenza, rhinovirus, RSV or coronavirus, amongst others.
- Even strep throat can resolve without treatment.
- Often gets better within 3 days (40% of patients) or at most a week (85%), though with infectious mononucleosis it can last two weeks.
- Less common causes are herpes simplex (primary infection), diphtheria, gonorrhoea and HIV.

Complications of strep throat include:
- quinsy (peritonsillar abscess)
- scarlet fever
- rheumatic fever
- glomerulonephritis
- flare of guttate psoriasis.

What useful questions could you ask Sanjiv at this stage? Write down at least three.

- 'Have you had a **fever**?' Fever is more likely to suggest strep.
- 'Do you have a **cough**?'
- 'Has your voice been **hoarse**?' Like cough, hoarseness in the presence of sore throat is more likely to signify viral infection.
- 'Have you had sore throats in the past?' or 'Tell me why you'd like antibiotics' may reveal more about the patient's **ICE**. As most people with sore throat don't see their doctor, you could also ask why he came at this time.

Sanjiv has not taken his temperature, but does not think he's had any fever. He has no cough and has not been hoarse. About two years ago he had a sore throat. It went away with the Strepsils his mother gave him. This time he'd like antibiotics because his sister has just had a baby and he really doesn't want the baby to catch anything.

Do you examine Sanjiv?

Yes. While the history is clear and straightforward, you may gain valuable added information from examining him, and it should not take long.

What do you examine?

- Take his pulse and temperature.
- Examine his throat (unless there are any symptoms or signs of epiglottitis).
- Check for cervical lymph nodes.
- Check the eardrums.
- Listen to the chest.
- Consider BP as it has not been taken for some time.
- You could also consider pulse oximetry.

Tip

Epiglottitis is a contraindication to examination of the throat as it can precipitate **laryngeal obstruction**. Symptoms of epiglottitis include:

► severe sore throat
► trouble breathing (often sitting forward)
► drooling
► dysphagia.

You find that Sanjiv's temperature is normal, pulse 76, and BP 128/65. His chest and TMs are normal. His throat is red (raw meat comes to mind). There are a few tender enlarged lymph nodes below the angle of jaw.

What do you do now?

(a) Prescribe antibiotics?
(b) Recommend simple measures only?
(c) Do a throat swab?

The right course of action is not obvious here and you could use additional help. The **Centor criteria** go back more than 30 years and were formulated for emergency room use, but can still be a valuable clinical tool (see Resources). They combine points from the history and examination to determine the likelihood of group B strep infection in adults. The patient gets one point for each of these:

- presence of tonsillar exudate
- presence of anterior cervical lymphadenopathy
- history of fever
- absence of cough.

If the Centor score is 3 or 4, it's likely to be strep. If it is 0 or 1, it's much less likely. The criteria are more useful for ruling strep out than for ruling it in.

Using Centor, Sanjiv scores 2, so the right course of action is still not clear-cut.

Swabbing his throat may be helpful here, though throat swabs are not now recommended as routine in general practice.

Going back to the question of management, either (a) or (c) would be appropriate here. For a patient happy with simple OTC measures, (b) would not be wrong.

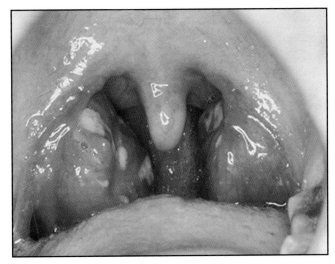

Figure 48.1   Tonsillitis with exudate.

Source: Reproduced with kind permission of Rila Publications Ltd, London.

On many occasions, a **delayed prescription** is suitable, along with the advice to use simple symptomatic relief alone for the next 24–48 hours and only get the prescription dispensed if symptoms persist.

In the end you decide to give antibiotics and swab his throat, asking him to ring in 3 days for the result. You tell him you're not sure antibiotics are necessary, but you think they're the best option for him at the moment.

What might you prescribe here?

Penicillin V (phenoxymethylpenicillin) is the drug of choice for strep throat. Give 500 mg qds for 10 days for an adult. For someone allergic to penicillin, erythromycin or another macrolide is suitable.

Sanjiv is happy with the prescription, though surprised he needs to take it for 10 days. He thanks you and says he's pleased he won't be giving his sore throat to his little niece.

Is there anything for you to add?

If Sanjiv has a non-streptococcal infection, he could still pass that on to his sister's baby. You should therefore advise him to keep away from his niece as much as possible until his throat is better. As a general piece of advice, handwashing is a good precaution before handling babies.

There's also value in giving him a patient information sheet on sore throat, so that he does not expect antibiotics on every future occasion.

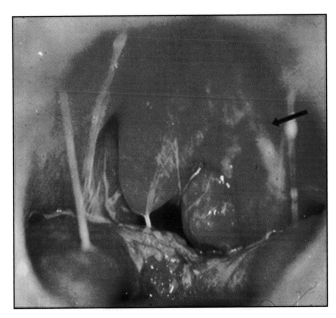

Figure 48.2   Quinsy.

Source: Reproduced with kind permission of Rila Publications Ltd, London.

Some sore throats need **urgent admission:**

- ► stridor
- ► difficulty breathing
- suspected epiglottitis
- suspected diphtheria or Stevens–Johnson syndrome
- possible Kawasaki disease.

CKS/NICE guidance recommend **urgent referral** for:

- suspected head or neck cancer
- sore throat lasting more than three weeks
- exudate or ulceration for more than three weeks
- dysphagia for more than three weeks.

Resources

SIGN: Management of sore throat and indications for tonsillectomy.

http://www.sign.ac.uk/pdf/qrg117.pdf

CKS/NICE: Sore throat – acute.

http://cks.nice.org.uk/sore-throat-acute#!topicsummary

Liverpool Medics: Clinical calculators – Centor criteria (modified).

http://liverpoolmedics.com/clinicalcalculator/centor_criteria.php

Centor RM, *et al.* The diagnosis of strep throat in adults in the emergency room. *Med Decis Making* 1981; 1(3): 239–246.

http://www.ncbi.nlm.nih.gov/pubmed/6763125

CASE

49 I'm tired all the time

Karen Phillips, age 55 years

Works in human resources

PMH: varicose veins; tattoo removal; benign breast lump; impaired GTT

Medication: nil

Karen Phillips sits down with a sigh and says she's tired literally all the time. She works full time, and her partner, with whom she lives, works abroad a lot. They have a dog and now she has to do all the walking as well as everything round the house. She admits she is rather house-proud.

You ask conversationally if her partner does his share of dog care and housework when he is home. She replies crisply that her partner is female, and no, Sue doesn't do that much.

Tip

Listen carefully to patients and beware of making assumptions.

You apologize, and she appears to overlook your mistake. 'Anyway I think it's all down to stress, but I thought I should check,' she finishes.

What single most useful question should you ask now?

Clarify her symptom with a question like 'What do you mean by tired?'

Tip

Be careful how you interpret symptoms too. 'Tired' can mean muscular weakness, daytime sleepiness, or lack of energy.

Karen means she has no energy. It's worse at the end of the day, though in fact she's tired pretty much as soon as she gets to her desk. This has been the case for about six months, since Sue got that new job which takes her all over Europe.

What further questions would you like to ask now? Write down at least six.

- 'Have you **lost weight**?' ► Unintentional weight loss is very significant.
- 'Do you have a **fever**? Or **night sweats**?' ► Fever and/or night sweats are also red flag symptoms.
- 'Do you have any **other symptoms**?' If necessary, prompt Karen by mentioning cough, pain, bowel habit, lumps anywhere.
- 'Have you **travelled abroad** in the last six months?'
- 'When was your last **period**?' The menopause can be linked with fatigue, as can early and late pregnancy.
- 'Are you **vegetarian**?' Many vegetarians manage to avoid anaemia, but vegans can run short of B12.
- 'What's your **mood** like? Do you feel low, or tearful? What things do you enjoy doing?' Depression is a very common cause of feeling tired all the time.
- 'What else has changed in your life?'

Karen says there are no other symptoms apart from aching knees and ankles after a long walk. Her weight is a steady 64 kg and she has no fever or night sweats. She went through the menopause four years ago. She eats meat, when she can be bothered to cook. As for foreign travel, she says, 'No such luck.' Work has got busier. She doesn't enjoy it like she used to, but there are plenty of things she does enjoy, like gardening and reading.

Some causes of being 'tired all the time'

There isn't a comprehensive list, but consider these conditions.

Social/situational
- Stress (home, work or both).
- Over-exercising.
- Lack of sleep.
- Dieting.

Mental health problems
- Depression.
- Anxiety.
- Anorexia.

Poisons
- Alcohol abuse.
- Illicit drugs.
- Prescribed drugs (e.g. betablockers, sedatives).
- Heavy metal poisoning (e.g. lead).

Infections
- Infectious mononucleosis.
- Hepatitis.
- HIV.
- TB.
- Bacterial endocarditis.
- Parasitic infections.

Endocrine
- Thyroid disease (over- or under-active).
- Diabetes.
- Cushing's.
- Pregnancy.
- Menopause.
- Hypogonadism.

Hypoxic
- Sleep apnoea.
- Anaemia (any type, but iron deficiency is common in women).
- Respiratory disease (e.g. COPD, asthma).
- Heart failure/myocardial insufficiency.

Chronic disease
- Renal disease.
- Liver disease.
- IBD.
- Coeliac disease.
- Almost any chronic disease (e.g. inflammatory arthritis).
- Chronic pain.

General Practice Cases at a Glance, First Edition. Carol Cooper and Martin L Block. © 2017 John Wiley & Sons, Ltd. Published 2017 by John Wiley & Sons, Ltd.

Malignant disease
- Cancer almost anywhere (especially metastatic).
- Lymphoma.
- Leukaemia.

Neurological
- Chronic fatigue syndrome.
- MS.

Should you examine her?

Yes. It is unlikely to be very helpful, but it may reveal something unexpected. Examination can also be useful for reassurance for both you and the patient. Anyone can get information from books or online, but only doctors (and some other health professionals) perform clinical examination.

What might you examine in particular? Make a list.

- Weight, BP and pulse, especially for arrhythmia.
- Conjunctivae for clinical anaemia.
- Chest for wheeze or other signs.
- Heart for murmur.
- Abdomen for masses or tenderness.
- Lymph nodes for evidence of infection or lymphoma.
- Thyroid for goitre, and signs of thyroid disease.
- Legs. She complains of aching knees and ankles, so this might be useful.

Her BP is 130/68, her weight is 65 kg, and her pulse is regular. You find nothing abnormal except for bilateral valgus ankles, which may account for her aching.

What do you do now?

As there are no red flags here, time is on your side. However, consider the value of a **blood test** to check for anaemia, diabetes (in view of her previous impaired glucose tolerance), thyroid function (thyroid disease can have few clinical signs), HIV (depending on level of risk) and coeliac disease.

You decide to request FBC, CRP, ferritin, folate, B12, U&Es, LFTs, TFTs and HbA1c, and ask to see her again in two weeks. Meanwhile you suggest to Karen that she paces herself, makes more time for herself, and makes sure she eats properly. When you extol the benefits of regular exercise, she reminds you that she walks a rather large Weimaraner twice a day. You apologize for having forgotten.

Karen returns in three weeks and reports that she feels much better. 'So it was just stress', she says. She has stopped doing things like ironing tea-towels and vacuuming daily, in favour of more 'me-time'. She has not yet got around to having those blood tests, but she got herself some more supportive trainers to wear when dog-walking, and has taken up mindfulness. 'You might benefit from it too, doctor', she adds with a smile.

How do you respond?

'Thank you', is a suitable reply. GPs do sometimes learn things from patients that they had not expected.

Do also remind her to have that blood test to check for diabetes. It would be prudent to 'safety-net' and ask her to return if her symptoms come back.

Resources

CKS/NICE Tiredness/fatigue in adults.
   http://cks.nice.org.uk/tirednessfatigue-in-adults
Be Mindful - from the Mental Health Foundation.
   http://bemindful.co.uk/
You might like to try Case 34: 'I seem to have lost weight'.

CASE

50 I'm worried about this lump, doctor

Alan Baxter, age 49 years

Dustman

PMH: Down's syndrome; mild learning disability; hypothyroidism

Medication: levothyroxine 100 μg daily

Alan Baxter is booked in to see you in a routine appointment. You know Alan and his sister Jane Baxter well. Alan has Down's syndrome and a mild learning difficulty.

He has kept well over the years and mainly sees you for routine illnesses. He lives at home with his older sister Jane, who has been Alan's carer for as long as you have known them both. They each have part time jobs, Alan working as a dustman. You usually see Alan in the company of his sister but today he is seeing you on his own. He is chatty walking down the corridor, talking about the weather and the football, and he sits down in your room.

What is a learning disability?

Around 1.5 m people in the UK have a learning disability. This can be mild, moderate or severe. A learning disability affects cognition and communication. This means they may struggle to:
- understand new or complex information
- learn new skills
- cope independently.

Causes
- genetic (e.g. Down's syndrome or Turner's syndrome)
- uterine (e.g. cerebral palsy, maternal illness in pregnancy)
- illness or brain injury in childhood (e.g. meningitis)
- neglect in early life
- untreated neonatal hypothyroidism.

You ask Alan what you can do for him and he tells you, 'I'm worried about this lump, doctor.'

What is your next question?

Start with a clear open question, something like, 'Tell me more about the lump.'

Alan goes on to say, 'I have a lump in my testicle. I'm worried about it.' He then stops talking and looks up expectantly to you.

What is the cue here and how will you explore it?

Alan has given you a verbal (and possibly non-verbal) cue to indicate that he is worried about his lump. You have two choices, either to address this now or to 'park' it and return at a later stage in the consultation. If you are to explore it now then ask a simple question such as, 'Tell me what you are worried about.'

You elect to explore his concerns now and Alan replies, 'I'm worried it might be cancer, doctor.' You thank Alan for sharing this information with you and offer a simple signposting comment.

What clear statement could signpost for Alan what you will do next?

A good signposting statement would be, 'Alan, I'm going to ask you a few more questions to find out more about this lump.'

What is a signpost?

Roger Neighbour, in his book *The Inner Consultation*, discusses signposts that mark the way in a consultation. They can provide some structure and clarity for patients.

In this case, you have recognized Alan's concerns and are informing him of the next part of the consultation. Signposts can be useful in any consultation, particularly if there is a degree of cognitive impairment and in consultations with young children.

What other questions would you ask now? Think of three.

- **How long** has the lump been present?
- Is it **painful**?
- Any **other symptoms**?
- Any **trauma**?

Alan tells you that it has been going on for a few weeks now. It isn't painful and there aren't any other symptoms. There is no history of any injury.

You decide you would like to examine him. You signpost this by saying, 'I would like to now examine the testes to see what's going on here.'

What else should you do before examination?

You should offer a chaperone to any male or female patients before undertaking a genital examination. Alan makes light of your offer, and shows you exactly where the lump is. Alan has a firm lump attached to the body of his left testis. There are no other scrotal abnormalities and there is no pain or tenderness.

What is the likely diagnosis?

This is likely to be a testicular tumour and as such needs prompt attention.

How do you manage this now?

▶ A new testicular lump always needs to be taken seriously. Alan needs urgent referral under the urgent cancer pathway and should be seen within two weeks, as recommended by NICE Guidance.

How would you communicate this to Alan?

As always, but especially so here, your communication should be clear and jargon-free, and give your patient the opportunity to ask any questions. You tell Alan that you think that he might be right, and that you would like to send him to a hospital clinic to see if the lump in the testicle is a cancer or something else. Alan looks a little worried and you ask him if there's anything he would like to ask. Alan asks if 'it is serious' to which you reply that you are taking it seriously and that he will be seen very soon in clinic (within two weeks) to get an answer.

General Practice Cases at a Glance, First Edition. Carol Cooper and Martin L Block. © 2017 John Wiley & Sons, Ltd. Published 2017 by John Wiley & Sons, Ltd.

How does competence fit into this consultation?

For an individual to have competence to make decisions about their care, you as a clinician must be confident in the patient's competence to make this decision. If this is not the case, it is good to involve the family and carers. In this case your patient should be able to:

- understand the **information**
- be able to understand and **make a decision** about the proposed management.

You have a sense that Alan has understood what you have told him and is able to understand the information you have shared about the proposed management. You check this with him, by asking him to run through what his understanding of the problem and the plan. Alan says 'I've got a lump in my testicle and you think it might be cancer, so I need to go to the clinic to see what is going on.' You confirm this with Alan.

Finally, what else could you offer Alan in the way of health promotion?

Anyone over 14 with a learning difficulty can have an annual health check with their GP. He should also have his TFTs checked at least once a year.

Although something for another day, Alan can be offered a health check appointment with the practice nurse. This would include baseline bloods (U+E, lipid profile, HbA1c, FBC), BP, BMI, cardiovascular risk assessment and general health promotion advice.

Alan thanks you for helping him today.

Resources

Royal College of General Practitioners, Clinical Resoures – Learning Disabilities.
http://www.rcgp.org.uk/learningdisabilities
Neighbour R. *The Inner Consultation*. 2nd edn. Oxford: Radcliffe Publishing, 2004.
The National Institute for Health and Clinical Excellence guideline Referral guidelines for suspected cancer: urological cancer (NICE, 2005).
Down's Syndrome Association.
http://www.downs-syndrome.org.uk/

You may also like to try Case 21: 'I'm fed up with my spots'.

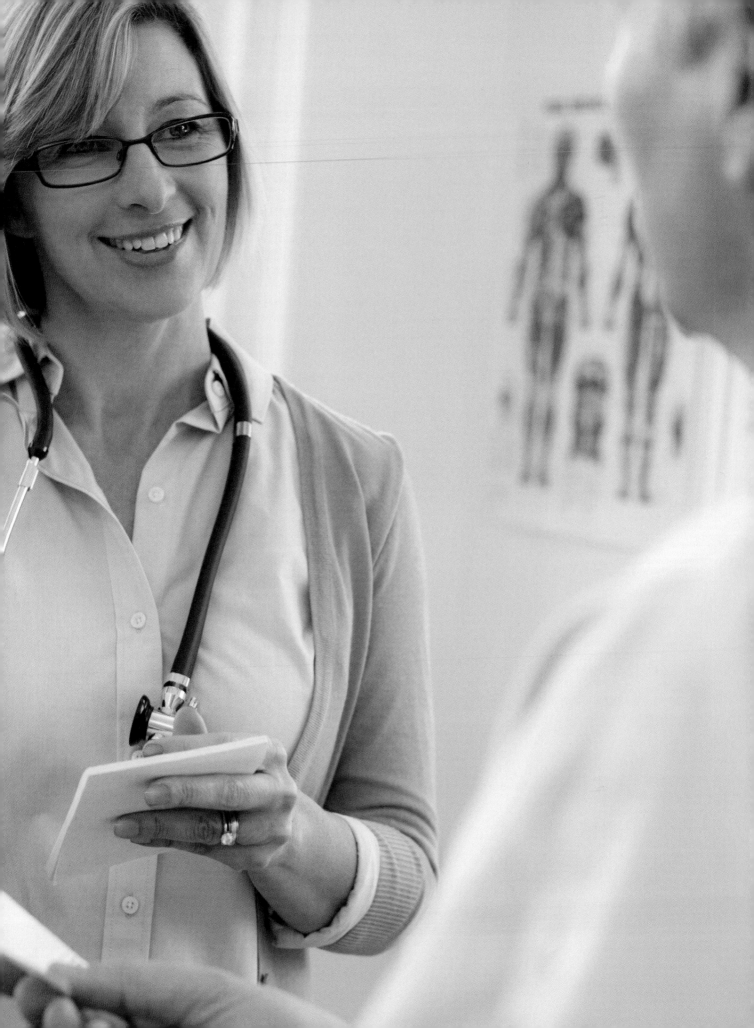

List of abbreviations

A&E	accident and emergency department		HDL	high density lipoprotein
ABPI	ankle branchial pressure index		HIB	*Haemophilus influenzae* type b
ADHD	attention deficit hyperactivity disorder		HIV	human immunodeficiency virus
BCC	basal cell carcinoma		HPV	human papilloma virus
bd	twice daily		HRT	hormone replacement therapy
BMI	body mass index		HVS	high vaginal swab
BNF	British National Formulary		IBD	inflammatory bowel disease
BP	blood pressure		IBS	irritable bowel syndrome
BPH	benign prostatic hyperplasia		IUS	intrauterine device
BTS	British Thoracic Society		LARC	long-acting reversible contraception
CBT	cognitive behavioural therapy		LDL	low density lipoprotein
CKS	Clinical Knowledge Summaries		LFT	liver function test
CMHT	Community Mental Health Team		LH	luteinising hormone
CNS	central nervous system		LMP	last menstrual period
COCP	combined oral contraceptive pill		MMR	measles, mumps and rubella
COPD	chronic obstructive pulmonary disease		MSU	mid stream urine (test)
CRP	C-reactive protein		NICE	National Institute for Clinical Excellence
CT	computerized tomography		NSAID	non-steroidal anti-inflammatory drug
CVD	cardiac vascular disease		PCOS	polycystic ovary syndrome
DEXA	dual energy X-ray absorptiometry		PEFR	peak expiratory flow rate
DJD	degenerative joint disease		PMH	past medical history
DRE	digital rectal examination		PPI	proton pump inhibitor
DVLA	Driver and Vehicle Licensing Agency		PSA	prostate specific antigen
DVT	deep vein thrombosis		RSI	repetitive strain injury
ECG	electrocardiography/electrocardiogram		RSV	respiratory syncytial virus
ED	erectile dysfunction		SNRI	selective noradrenaline reuptake inhibitor
EFGR	estimated glomerular filtration rate		SSRI	selective serotonin reuptake inhibitor
ESR	erythrocyte sedimentation rate		STI	sexually transmitted infection
FB	foreign body		TB	tuberculosis
FBC	full blood count		TFT	thyroid function test
FGM	female genital mutilation		TOP	termination of pregnancy
FH	family history		TSH	thyroid stimulating hormone
FSH	follicle-stimulating hormone		U&E	urea and electrolytes
GGT	gamma-glutamyl transpeptidase		URTI	upper respiratory tract infection
GORD	gastro-oesophageal reflux disease		UTI	urinary tract infection
GUM	genito-urinary medicine			

General Practice Cases at a Glance, First Edition. Carol Cooper and Martin L Block. © 2017 John Wiley & Sons, Ltd. Published 2017 by John Wiley & Sons, Ltd.

Index of cases by speciality

Cardiovascular problems: Cases 11, 26, 31, 40
Care of the elderly: Cases 8, 25, 30
Child health: Cases 1, 7, 12, 15, 29, 38, 43
Dermatology: Cases 21, 33, 43
Endocrine problems: Cases 9, 22, 42
End of life care: Case 36
Eyes and ENT: Cases 2, 13, 17, 20, 48
Gastrointestinal problems: Cases 10, 12, 32, 38, 41, 45
Mental health: Cases 2, 7, 14, 37, 44, 50
Men's health: Cases 18, 35, 50

Musculoskeletal problems: Cases 4, 8, 19, 47
Neurology: Cases 5, 17, 30
Respiratory problems: Cases 3, 28, 29, 36
Women's health: Cases 11, 23, 24, 27, 39, 46

Common general practice presentations

Headache: Case 5
Insomnia: Case 16
Tiredness: Case 49
Weight loss: Case 34

General Practice Cases at a Glance, First Edition. Carol Cooper and Martin L Block. © 2017 John Wiley & Sons, Ltd. Published 2017 by John Wiley & Sons, Ltd.

Index

abdominal pain, children   80–81
Abortion Act 1967   58
acid dyspepsia   93
acne   46–47
acute cough   12
acute limb ischaemia   85
addiction   33
Adult Safeguarding Team   23
afferent pupillary defect   38
alcohol, acid dyspepsia   93
alcohol abuse   33
alcohol detox   33
alcohol-induced pain   73
alcohol worker   33
allergic conjunctivitis   44
allergies   62
allodynia   41
amenorrhoea   11
anal carcinoma   26–27
anal fissure   26
analgesia   15, 97
analgesia over-use headache   16
anal pain   26–27
angiotensin-converting enzyme inhibitor (ACE inhibitor)   57
anorexia nervosa   10–11
antibiotics   31, 32, 45, 47, 55, 60, 98–99
anticoagulation   19
antidepressants   43, 92
anti-epileptics   43
antihistamines   91
antihypertensive medication   57
anxiety   78–79
anxiety disorders   78–79
arterial occlusion, acute   84, 85
asbestos exposure   12
asthma   62–63
atopic eczema   90–91
atrial fibrillation   18–19
attention deficit disorder (ADD)   20
attention deficit hyperactivity disorder (ADHD)   20–21
'atypical eating disorder'   10
aura, migraine   16
autism   20, 21
autistic spectrum disorder (ASD)   21

back pain   96–97
bedside manners   3
behavioural changes, dementia   64
berry aneurysm   17
binge-eating disorder   10
bladder symptoms   50
blepharitis   44
blood pressure   56–57
blood tests   25, 48–49, 69, 73, 101
BMI   24, 57
body language   2, 3
body mass index (BMI)   24, 57
boom and bust cycle   43
bowel habit changes   26
bowel malignancy   68

breast cancer   94–95
breast cancer family history clinic   94–95
breast-feeding   31
'B symptoms,' lymphoma   73
bulimia nervosa   10

caffeine   36, 37
calcium-channel blocker   19, 57
cancer, end of life care   76–77
Candida infection   52–53
capsaicin   43
cardiovascular problems   18–19, 28–29, 56–57, 84–85
cardioversion   19
care of the elderly   22–23, 54–55, 64–65
cases   7–103
cauda equina syndrome   97
Centor criteria, strep throat   98
CHA2DS2VASc   19
chest pain   60, 66–67
chest x-ray (CXR)   13, 19
child abuse   20, 35
child health
   ADHD   20–21
   asthma   62–63
   autism   20–21
   cough   62–63
   crying baby   34–35
   dehydration   30
   diarrhoea/vomiting   30–31
   fever   8–9
   immunizations   8, 9
   itch   90–91
   rashes   90
   tummy ache   80–81
   urinary tract infections   9
chlamydia   52
chronic cough   12
chronic limb ischaemia   84
chronic obstructive pulmonary disease (COPD)   12–13, 60–61
chronic pain   41–43
circulation, eating disorders   11
CKS/NICE guidelines   11, 73, 99
clinical decision-making tools   5
clinical reasoning   4–5
closed questions   2, 64
clotrimazole   52
cocaine, use in pregnancy   20, 21
colic   34
combined oral contraceptive pill (COCP)   47, 82–83
Community Mental Health Team (CMHT)   11
competence   47, 103
complex regional pain syndrome   41–42
concentration, children   20
confusion, acute   54–55
constipation   10, 26, 80
consultation   2–3
contact lenses   44, 82
contraceptive pill   82–83

COPD   12–13, 60–61
corticosteroids   60, 63, 91
cough   12–13, 62–63
crying, babies   34–35
Cry-Sis   35
cues   46, 102
Cushing's disease   24, 25
cycle of change   33

death certificate   77
definition phase, clinical reasoning   4, 5
dehydration   30, 86
dementia   64–65
depression   64, 79, 92, 100
dermatology   46–47, 70–71, 90–91
DESMOND programme   48, 88, 89
diabetes education program   40, 48, 88, 89
diabetes keto-acidosis   81
Diabetes UK   48, 88, 89
diagnosis   4–5
diarrhoea   30–31, 86–87
diazepam (Valium)   78
discharge, ear   32
donepezil   65
drinking, excessive   33
drug-induced conditions   24, 36

ear, nose and throat (ENT) cases   10–11, 32, 98–99
ear pain   32
eating disorders   10–11
eating disorders unit   11
ECG, atrial fibrillation   18
echocardiogram   19
EGFR (epithelial growth factor receptor) mutation   13
elder abuse   22–23
elderly, care of the   22–23, 54–55, 64–65
emergency ambulance   67
emollients   91
endocrine problems   24–25, 48–49, 88–89, 100
end of life care   76–77
ENT cases   10–11, 32, 98–99
epiglottis   98
erectile dysfunction   74–75
etonorgestrel implant   59
examination   3
   see also individual conditions
exercise   24, 37, 49, 57
eye pain   38–39
eye problems   38–39, 44–45

family history   3, 16, 21, 56, 94
family tree   94
feeling down   92
feet, thinking on   3
female genital mutilation (FGM)   28, 29
femoro-popliteal bypass   85
fever, children   8–9
fit note, back pain   97
focused history-taking   2–3

General Practice Cases at a Glance, First Edition. Carol Cooper and Martin L Block. © 2017 John Wiley & Sons, Ltd. Published 2017 by John Wiley & Sons, Ltd.

folic acid 28
FRAX tool 50
function 3

gastric malignancy 93
gastroenteritis, children 30–31
gastrointestinal problems 26–27, 68–69, 80–81, 86–87, 93
generalized anxiety disorder (GAD) 78
Gillick competence 47
glaucoma, acute 44
golden minute 2
gonorrhoea 52

haemoptysis 12
Hajj 82–83
hay fever 10–11
Hba1c levels 48–49, 75, 88
headache 16–17
health promotion 60–61, 103
health visitor 21, 34
healthy eating 88
hearing 32
Heberden's nodes 14, 15
hepatitis B 52–53
history-taking 2–3
    see also individual conditions
HIV test 52–53
hoarseness 98
Hodgkin's lymphoma 73
hormone replacement therapy (HRT) 50–51
hospital admission 11, 19, 60, 99
HRT 50–51
hyperactive/impulsive behaviour 20
hyperalgesia 41
hypertension 28, 29, 56–57
hyperventilation 79
hypogonadism 74
hypothetico-deductive model 5
hypothyroidism 24–25

ibuprofen 9
ideas, concerns and expectations (ICE) 3
imaging, knee pain 15
immunizations 8, 9, 83
inattention 20
infants, crying 34–35
infections 9, 30, 90, 91, 100
infective conjunctivitis 44–45
inflammatory arthritis 97
inhalers 60, 62–63
initial complaint 5
initiation stage, clinical reasoning 4, 5
insomnia 36–37
intermittent claudication 84
introductions 3
investigations/tests see individual conditions
irritable bowel syndrome (IBS) 68–69, 87
ischaemic heart disease 66–67
itch 90–91

Kawasaki disease 9
knee pain 14–15

laryngeal obstruction 98
learning disability 102–103
legal issues, dementia 65
leg pain 84–85
levator ani syndrome 26
levothyroxine 25
lifestyle measures 15, 56, 69, 75, 93

long-acting reversible contraception (LARC) 59
lower urinary tract symptoms (LUTS) 40
lubricants 50
lung cancer 12–13, 19, 76–77
lymph node enlargement 72, 73
lymphoma 72–73

malignant melanoma 70–71
management plan card, asthma 63
Marcus Gunn pupil 38
mechanical (non-specific) back pain 96
medical termination of pregnancy 58
medroxyprogesterone acetate 59
memory assessment test 65
memory clinic 65
memory impairment 64–65
meningococcal disease 8, 9
men's health 40, 74–75, 102–103
menstrual cycle see periods
mental health 10–11, 33, 78–79, 92, 102–103
metered dose inhaler 62
metformin 49
micro-suction 32
mifepristone 58
migraine 16–17, 81, 82
misoprostol 58
mole, changes in 70–71
multiple sclerosis 38–39
muscle power, eating disorders 11
musculoskeletal problems 14–15, 41–43, 96–97
myocardial infarction 66, 67

neck stiffness 16
nerve root pain (sciatica) 96, 97
neurogenic pain 84
neurological examination 38
neurology 16–17, 38–39, 64–65
neuropathic pain 41, 43
NHS Breast Screening Programme 95
NICE guidelines 11, 73, 99
night sweats 72, 73
non-blanching rash 9
non-Hodgkin's lymphoma 73
non-steroidal anti-inflammatory drugs (NSAIDs) 15, 43, 93
non-verbal cues 46
norethisterone 59, 82
notifiable diseases 30, 31

obesity 24
oestrogens 50–51
omeprazole 93
open questions 2, 64
opioids, chronic pain 43
optic neuritis 38
oral rehydration solution 31
osteoarthritis 14–15, 97
osteoporosis 50
otitis externa 32
otitis media 32
ovarian malignancy 68
overweight 24

pain
    in eczema 90, 91
    irritable bowel syndrome 68
    see also individual types
pain scores, knee pain 14
palliative care 76–77

panic attack 78
panic disorder 78–79
papilloedema 39
paracetamol 9, 15, 43
patient information leaflets 46, 48, 69, 79, 91, 99
patient's own diagnosis 5
pattern recognition 5
penicillin V (phenoxymethylpencillin) 99
people skills 3
periods 10, 24
    acne 46
    avoiding 82–83
peripheral vascular disease 84–85
peritoneal irritation 81
peritonism 80
persistent pain 41–43
persistent pain cycle 42
pertussis 62
pervasive developmental disorders (PDD) 21
phenoxymethylpencillin (penicillin V) 99
physiotherapy 15, 97
piles 26
place of death 76
polycystic ovary syndrome (PCOS) 24, 46
pre-diabetes 40, 75
pre-eclampsia 28–29
pregnancy 20, 21, 28–29, 58–59
'preventer' medication 63
previous medical history (PMH) 3
primary headaches 16
proctalgia fugax 26
prostaglandin 58
prostate cancer 40
prostate specific antigen (PSA) test 40
proteinuria 28, 29
proton pump inhibitors (PPI) 93
'6 Ps' 85
PSA test 40
psychological therapy 75, 78
psychosocial therapy 42
pulmonary rehabilitation 61

Qrisk calculator 57
question types 2, 64
quinsy 99

range of movement (ROM), knee pain 14
Rapid Response team 55
rashes 9, 90
rectal bleeding 26, 27
recurrent laryngeal nerve palsy 13
red eye 44–45
red flags 3, 5
    autism 21
    dehydration 30
    diarrhoea/vomiting, children 30
    febrile children 8
    low back pain assessment 96
    red eye 44
refinement, clinical reasoning 4, 5
reflection 5, 46
reflux 34
relapse prevention, alcohol abuse 33
relatives, degrees of 94
respiratory problems 12–13, 60–63, 76–77
resuscitation status 76
retinoids 47
ringworm 90

safety net 45, 61, 87
salbutamol 62

scabies   90
sciatica   96, 97
scleritis   44
SCOFF questionnaire   10
screening tools, dementia   65
seborrhoeic keratosis   71
sexually transmitted infections (STIs)   26, 51,
   52–52
shortness of breath   60–61
shoulder pain   22–23
sign-posting   3, 102
sildenafil   75
Six-item Cognitive Impairment Test
   (6-CIT)   65
sleep apnoea   36, 37
sleep hygiene   37
sleep problems   36–37
smoking   12, 49, 56, 57, 62, 93
social services   23
social worker   21
SOCRATES pain assessment   2, 66
sore throat   98–99
spirometry   13, 61
spot diagnosis   5
spots   46–47
SSRIs   92

statins   24, 49, 57
steroids   60, 63, 91
stomach, burning sensation   93
stomach cancer   93
stomach cramps   68–69
stool colour, infants   31
straight leg raise   96
strep throat   98
subarachnoid haemorrhage (SAH)   16, 17
subclinical hypothyroidism   25
subconjunctival haemorrhage   44
Sudeck's atrophy   41–42
suicide risk assessment   92
super-obesity   24
super-super-obesity   24
swinging light test   38, 39

tension-type headaches   16
termination of pregnancy   58–59
testicular lumps   72, 102–103
testicular tumor   102–103
thiamine   33
thrush   52–53
tiredness   54–55, 100–101
tonsillitis   81, 99
travel   12, 30

Trichomonas vaginalis   52
'tummy ache'   80–81
2-week wait referral criteria   27, 71, 87, 99,
   102
type 2 diabetes   48–49, 75, 88–89

UK Medical Eligibility Criteria (UKMEC) for
   the Oral Contraceptive   82
urinary tract infections (UTIs)   9, 54–55
uveitis   44

vaginal discharge   52–53
Valium (diazepam)   78
vegetarians   100
verbal cues   46, 102
viral infection   86
vitamin D   28
vomiting   17, 30–31

waist size   24
weight gain   24–25
weight loss   72–73, 100
wheeze   62
women's health   28–29, 50–53, 58–59, 82–83,
   94–95
worst-case scenario   5